The Big Beautiful Book of Burping, Belching, & Barfing

Jimmy Huston

Copyright © 2020 Jimmy Huston

ISBN: 978-1-970022-50-6

All rights reserved, including the right to use or reproduce this book or portions thereof in any form whatsoever without written permission from the publisher except in the case of brief quotations embodied in critical articles or reviews.

All images are used under license from Shutterstock.com

Cosworth Publishing
21545 Yucatan Avenue
Woodland Hills CA 91364
www.cosworthpublishing.com

For information regarding permission,
please send an email to office@cosworthpublishing.com.

Dedicated to

Pepto Bismol, Tumeez, Zofran, Dramamine, Nauzene, Emetrol, Kaopectate, & Ginger Ale

PART 1
BURPING

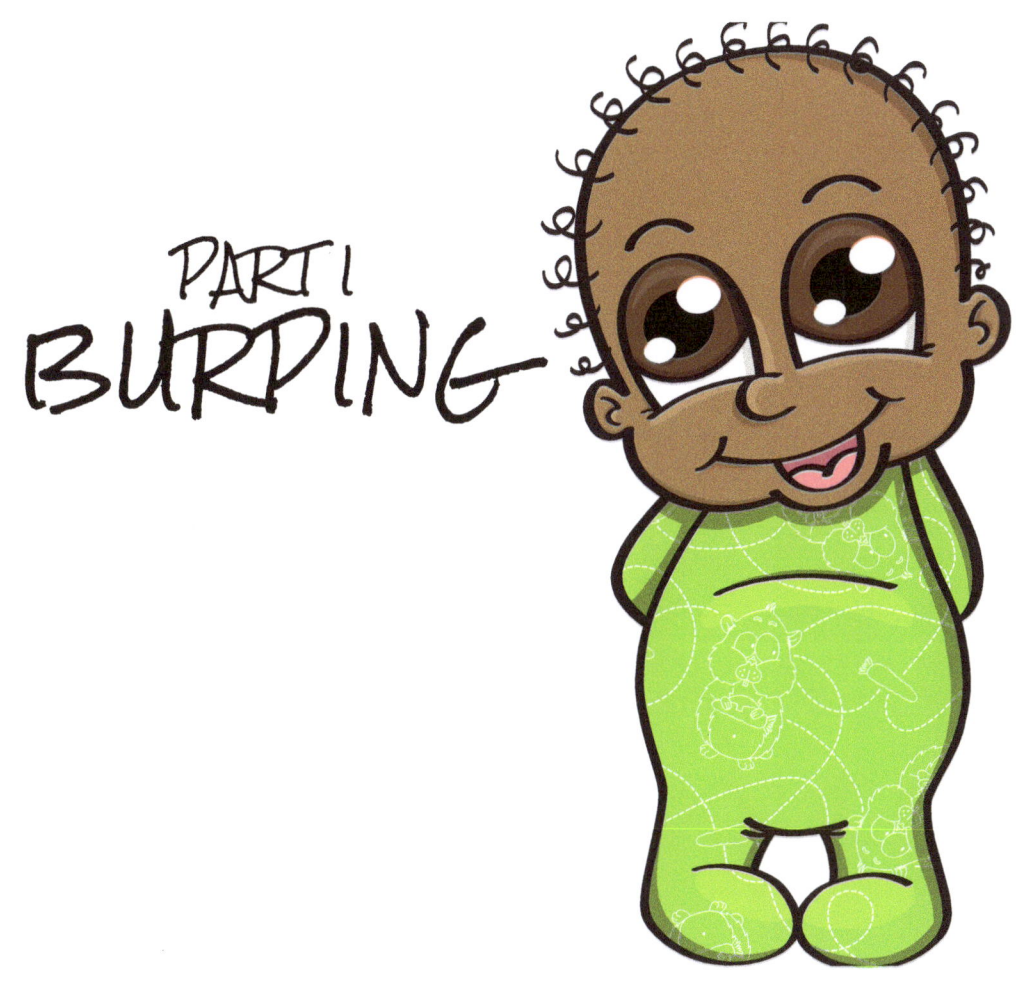

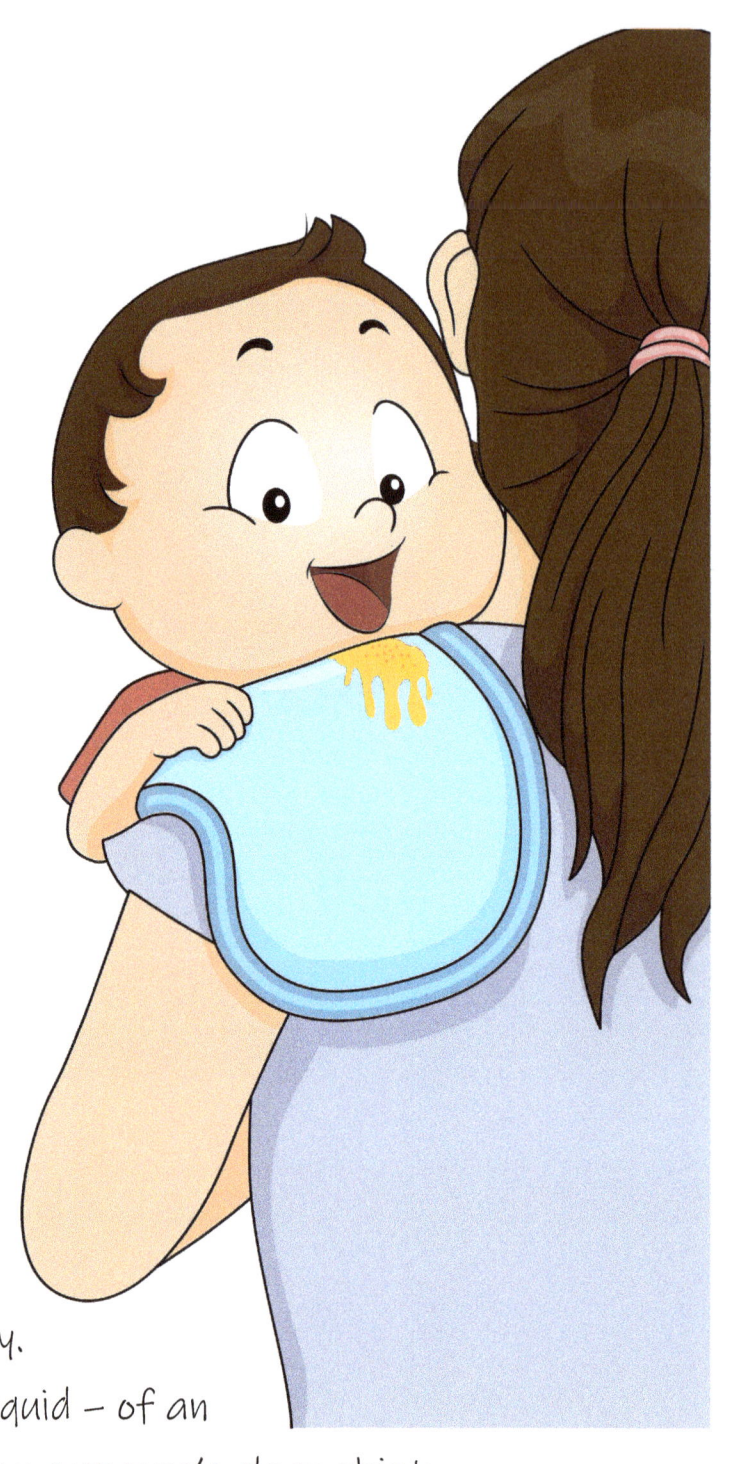

It was small and quiet.
Just a few tiny bubbles probably.
And a little bit of some sickish liquid – of an
uncertain color – that ended up on someone's clean shirt.

It's worth 10 points, just to get you started.

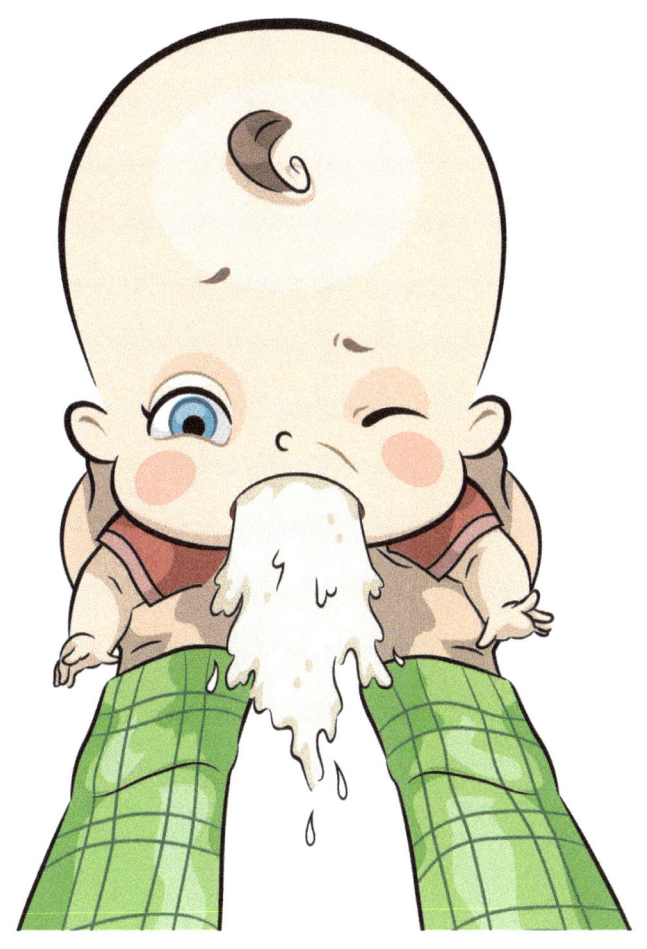

Even today, if you ask your mom about it, she'll both smile and grimace.
She may say she remembers it. She may not.
But she does.

5 POINTS IF SHE SMILES. 10 POINTS IF SHE GRIMACES.
25 POINTS IF SHE SAYS SHE REMEMBERS IT.
500 POINTS IF SHE KEPT THE STAINED GARMENT.

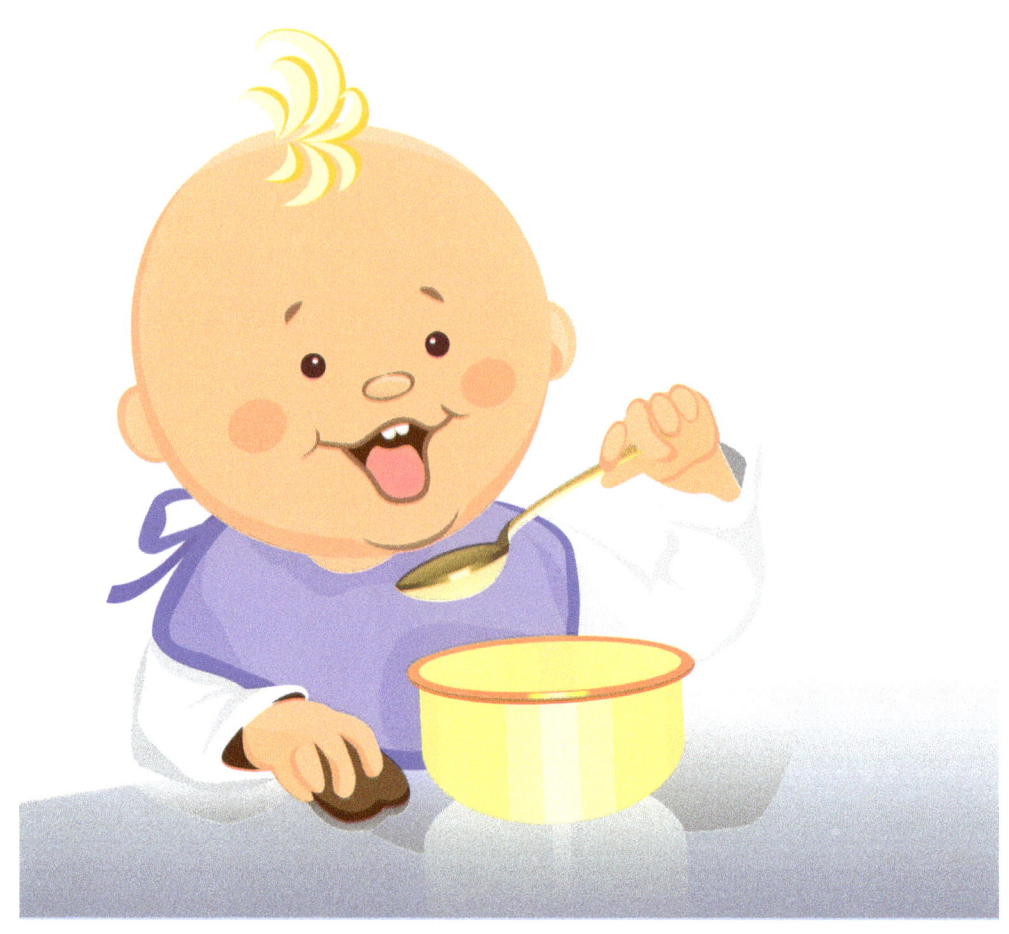

For a while your burps were cute. They were quiet and beyond your control. They just popped out. And that was okay, even with the big people.

In fact, they would put you over their shoulder and try to make you burp by patting your back.

So where did burping go wrong?

Well, after a while, your burps were boring.

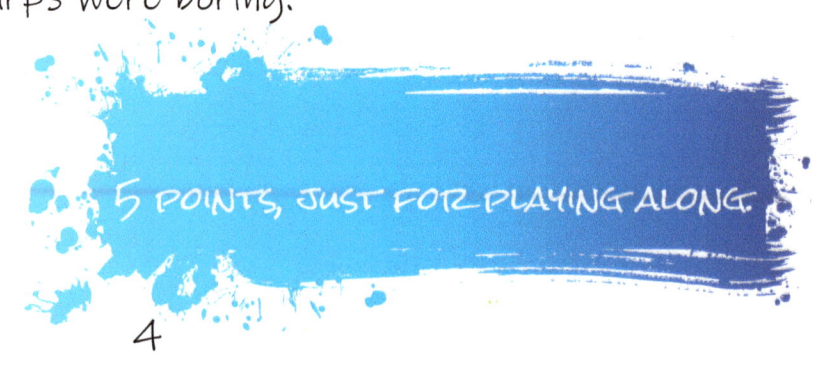

5 POINTS, JUST FOR PLAYING ALONG

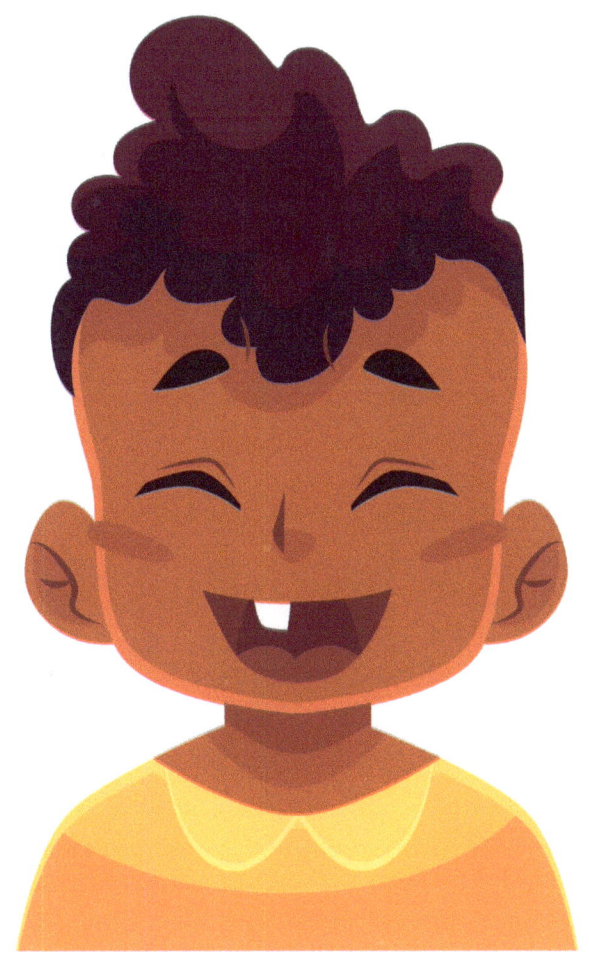

And you grew up.

Most burps just aren't that interesting.

That's because burps are controllable.

You know when they're coming — and you can let them out quietly — or you can announce them with a flourish. Or, sometimes, you just swallow them.

The polite thing to do is keep it quiet. A silent burp.

But what's the point if no one knows you're being polite?

For a burp to really count, it should be audible.

THAT MAKES IT WORTH 10 POINTS. TRY IT.

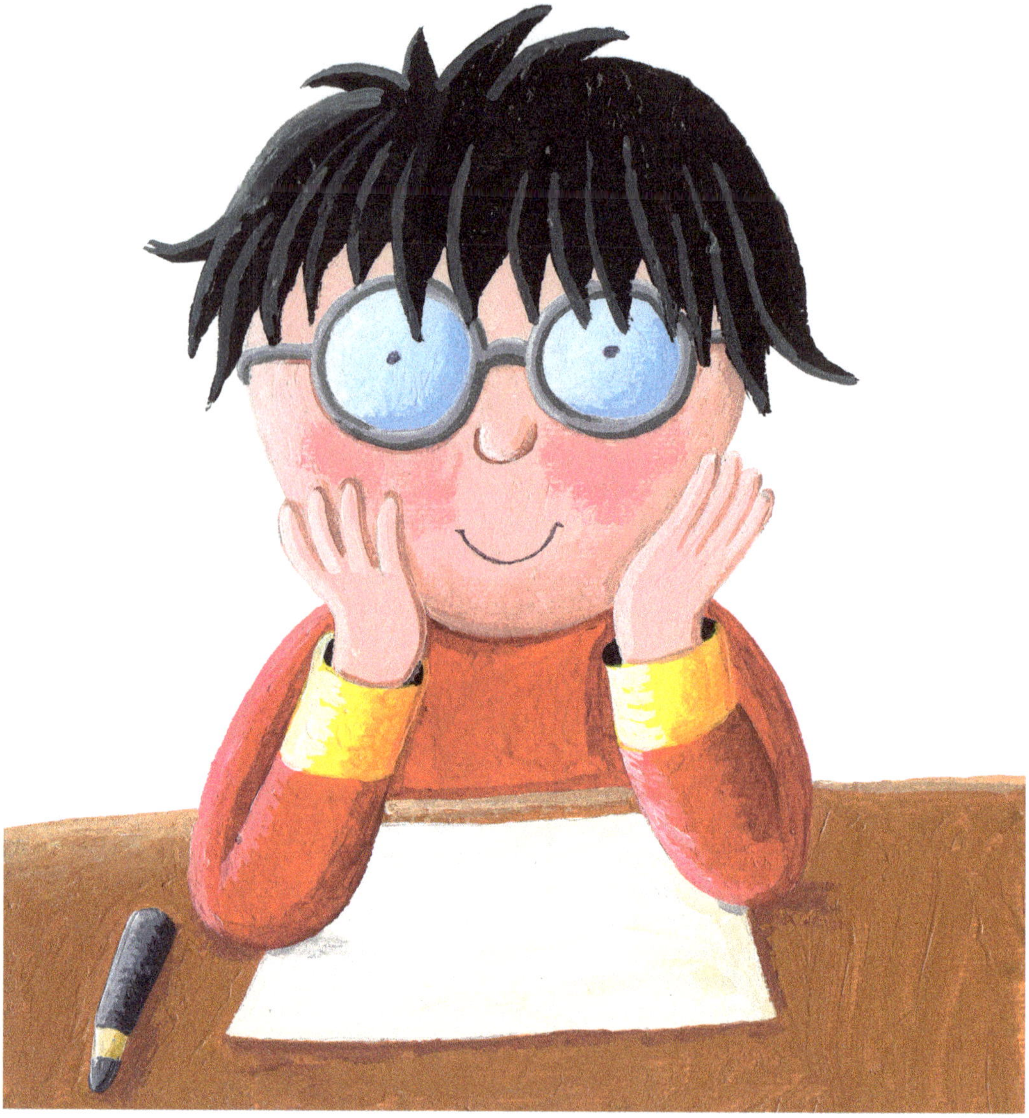

Swallowing a burp isn't the end of it.

You know it's coming back up, sooner or later. Usually it's a little stronger when it does. And the timing is usually worse.

A good burp will provide a little relief. Not much relief, but maybe a little bitty "aaaahhh..."

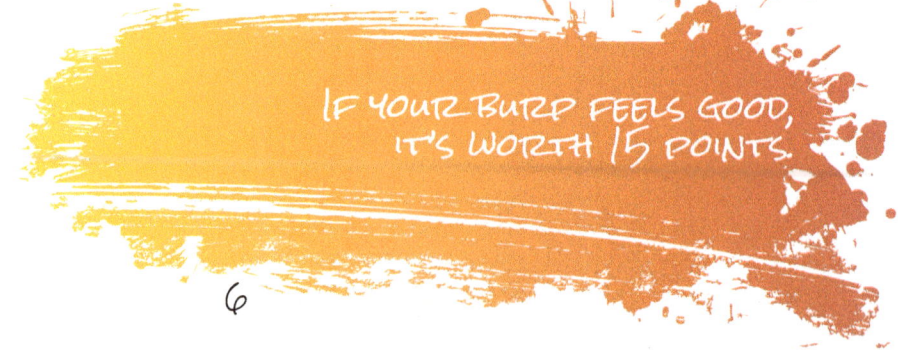

IF YOUR BURP FEELS GOOD, IT'S WORTH 15 POINTS.

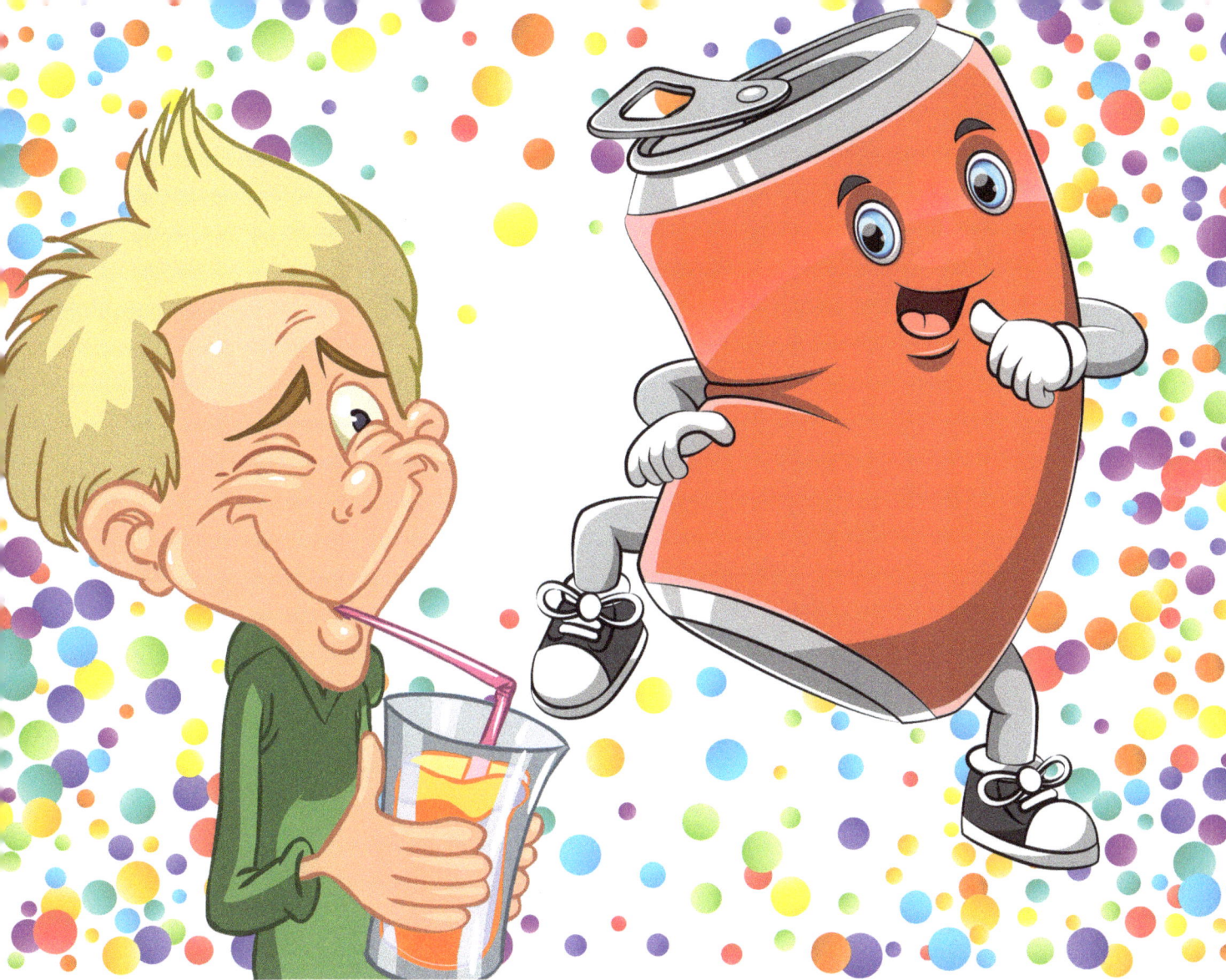

    For example, carbonation can make you burp. That's part of its charm. It can make you smile. That may make you want another sip, which probably means another burp. And so on.

    Sometimes a burp has company – a little something that bubbles up your throat and coats it with cootie juice. It's not usually too bad – just a little warning of what's possible. That's called "vurping."

    A fancier word for it is "eructing."

A LITTLE "COOTIE JUICE" IS WORTH 25 POINTS.

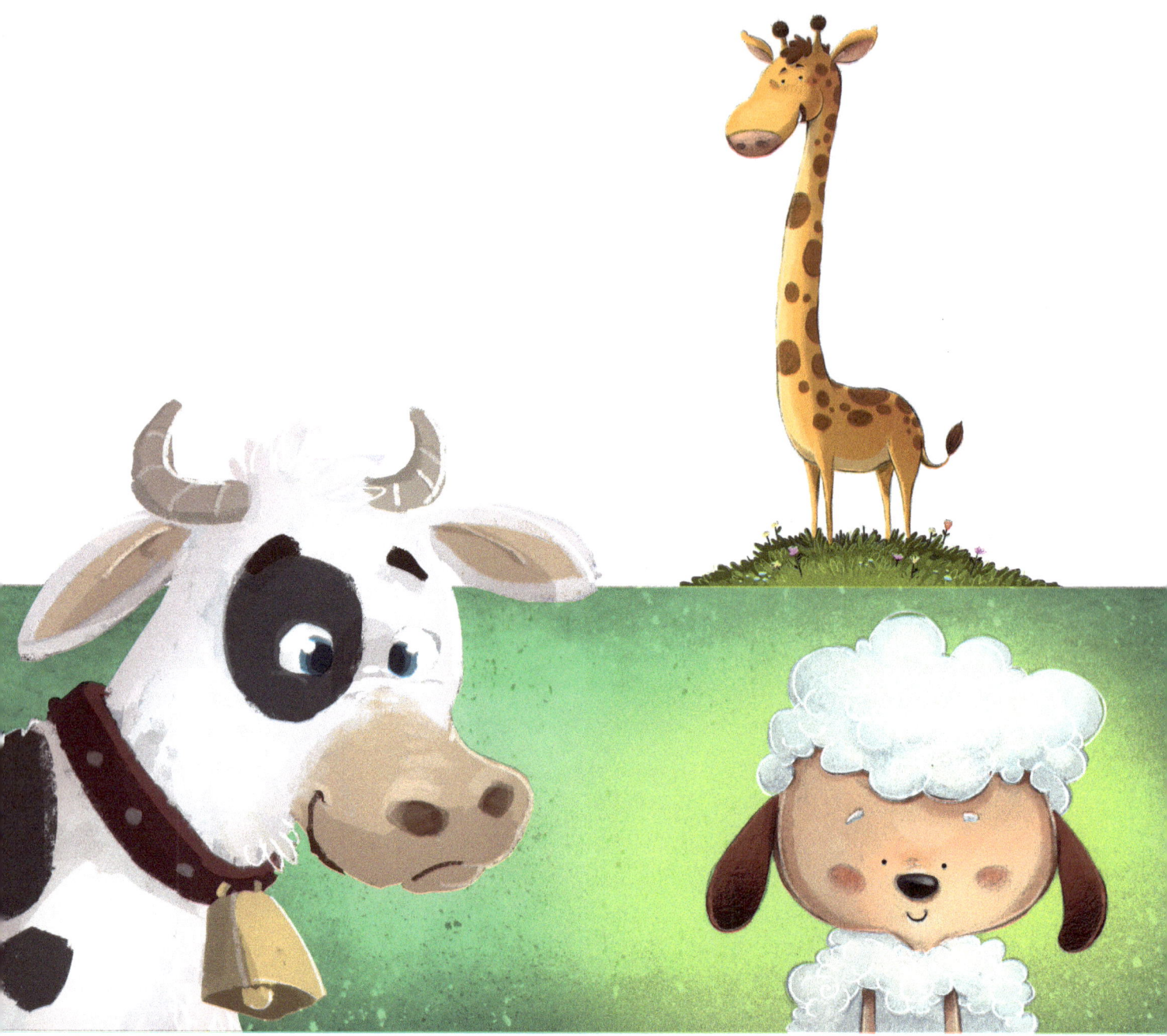

Cows burp. Goats, sheep, buffalo, giraffes, deer, elk, and camels burp. (They all burp up their food to chew it again — and are called "ruminant" animals.)

Your mom burps. Your doctor burps. Your minister burps — or your rabbi, priest, or mullah. It's okay to burp.

Usually.

IF YOU CATCH ANY ONE OF THEM BURPING, GIVE YOURSELF 100 POINTS. GIVE THEM 50 POINTS.

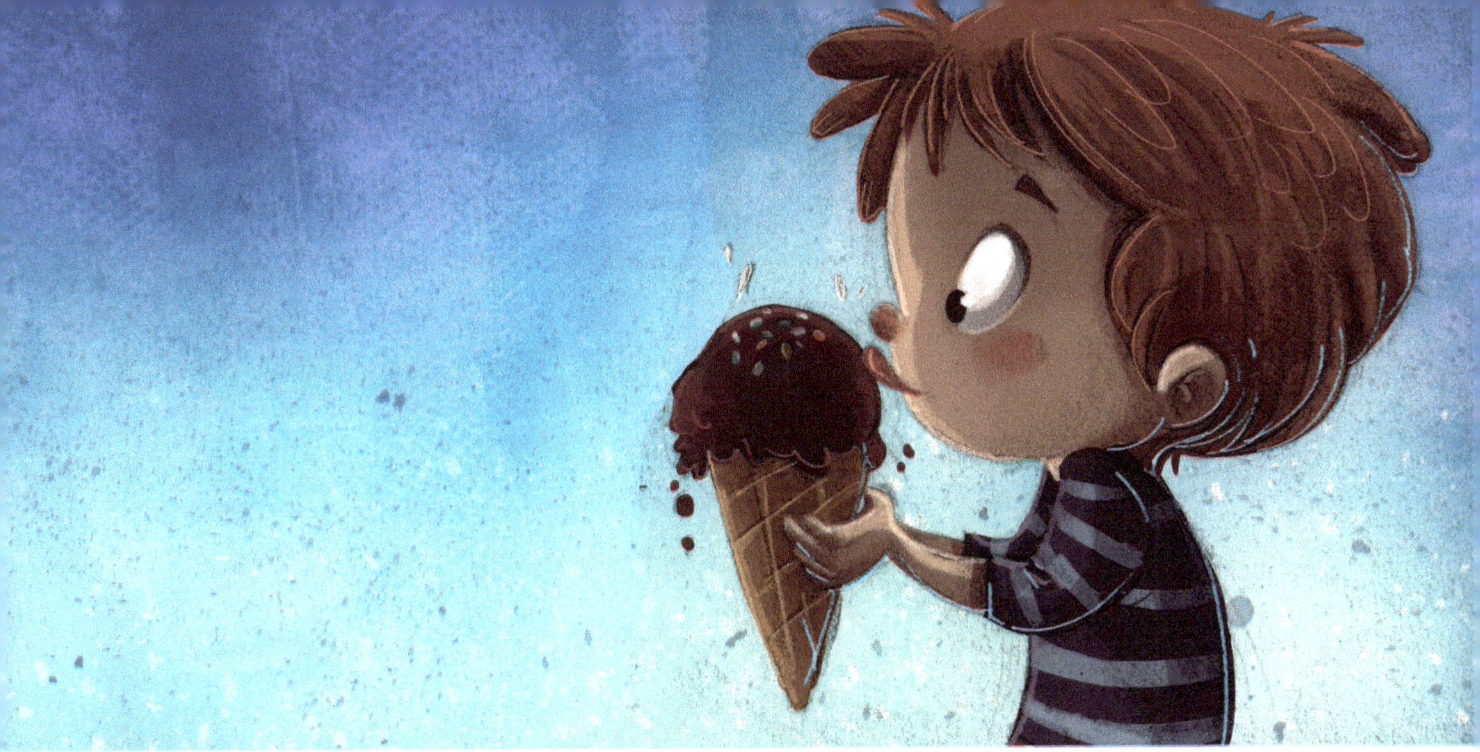

A really good burp can have a flavor. So can a bad burp. Yuk.

A burp usually tastes like whatever you just ate or drank. That's why it's better to eat ice cream than salad. You can explain that to your mom.

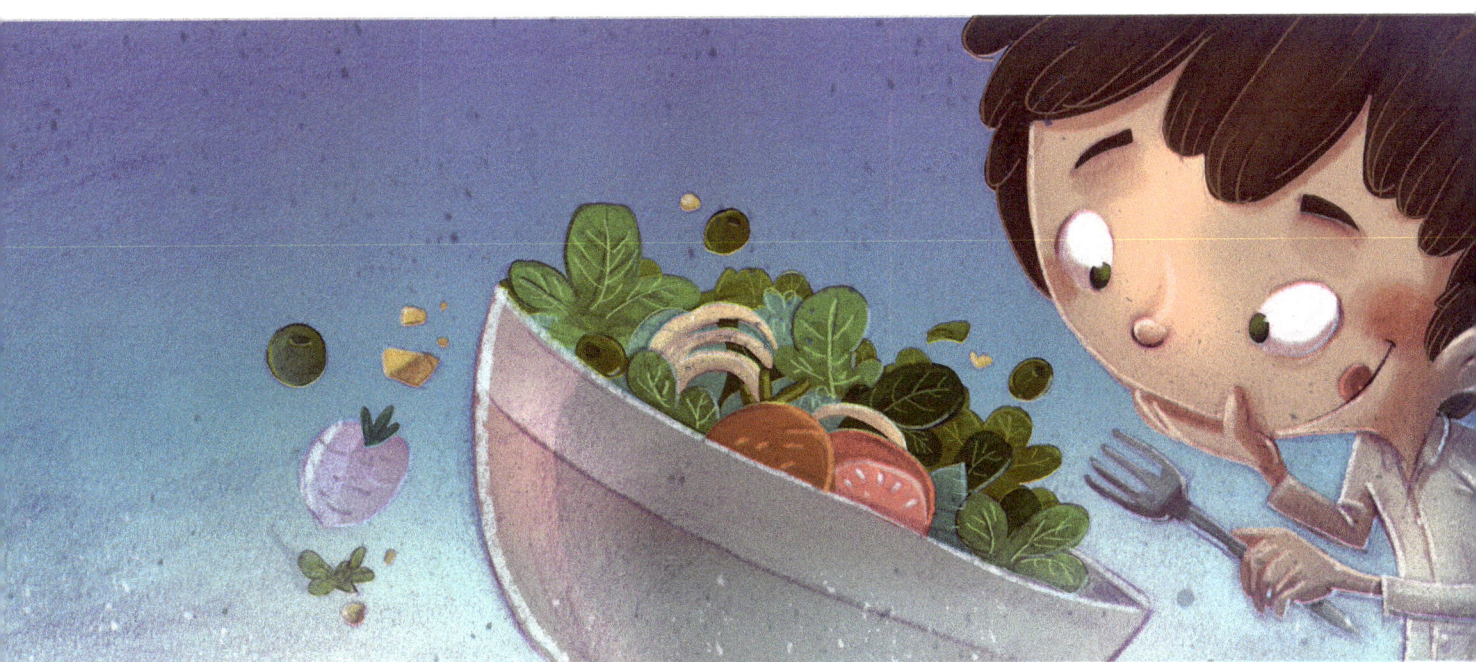

IF YOUR MOM BELIEVES YOU, THAT'S WORTH 500 POINTS. (AND YOU'LL GET ICE CREAM, TOO.)

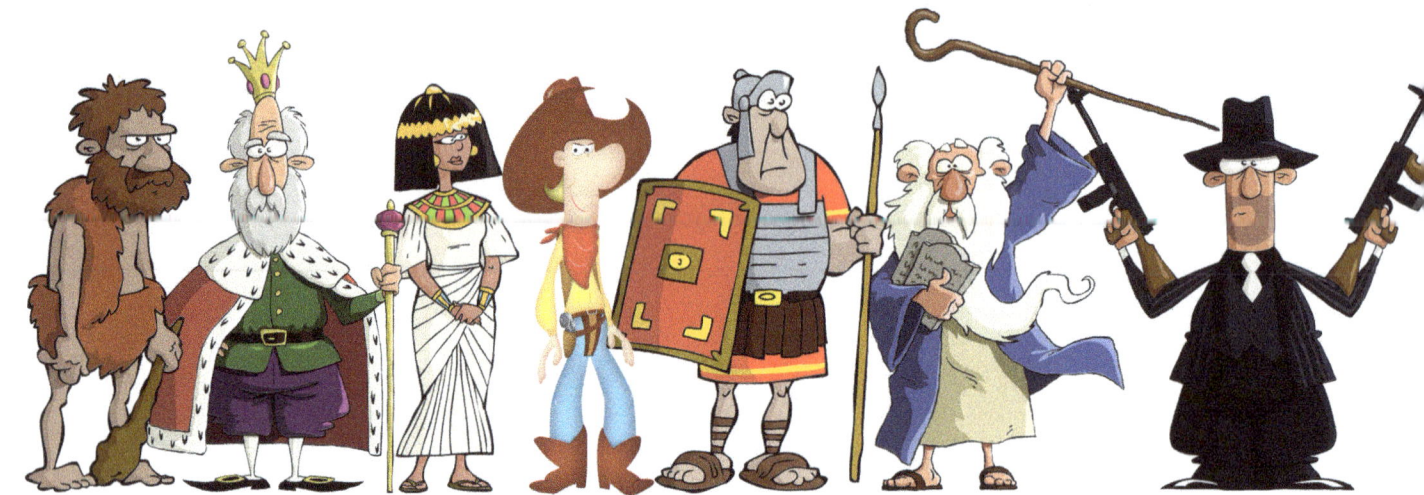

There's nothing new about burping. There's burping all through history. Peasants, soldiers, drunkards, and slobs all burped. But that's not all. Kings were famous for burping. And Vikings, too. And all the Popes. In fact, all of these people burped.

- Napoleon
- George Washington
- Billy the Kid
- Cleopatra
- Nelson Mandela
- Al Capone
- King Tut
- Gandhi

- Calamity Jane
- Genghis Kahn
- Harriet Tubman
- The Beatles
- William Shakespeare
- Helen Keller
- Buddah
- Michelangelo

If you don't know who all of these people are, you will.
Just remember that they're all burpers.

WHEN YOUR TEACHER MENTIONS THESE PEOPLE, TELL HER THAT THEY BURPED. THAT'S WORTH 300 POINTS.

PART II
THE BELCH

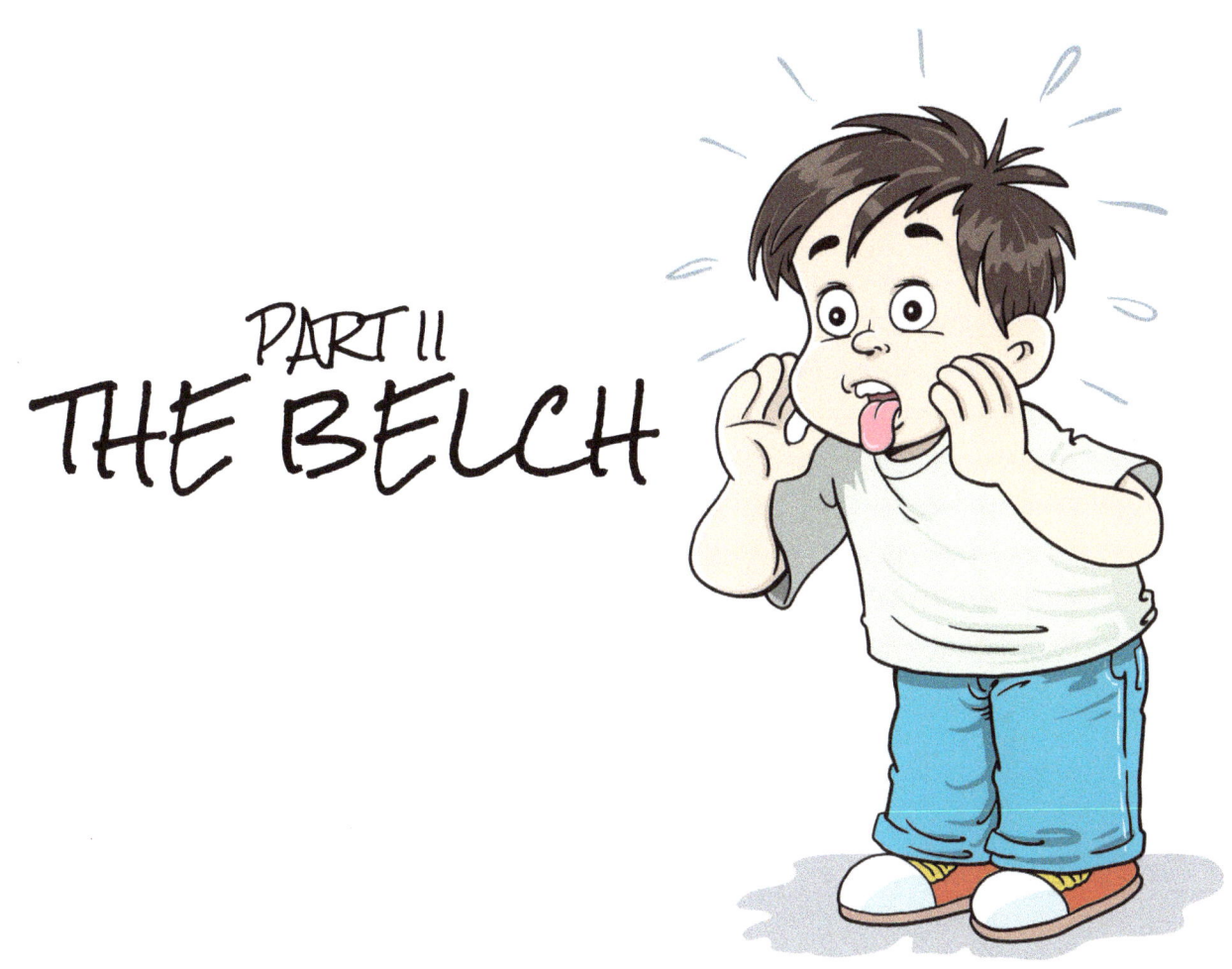

Belches are a little like burps, but there's one big difference.

It's not that they're bigger. But they may be.

It's not that they're louder. But they may be.

The difference between a big ol' burp and a satisfying belch is simple.

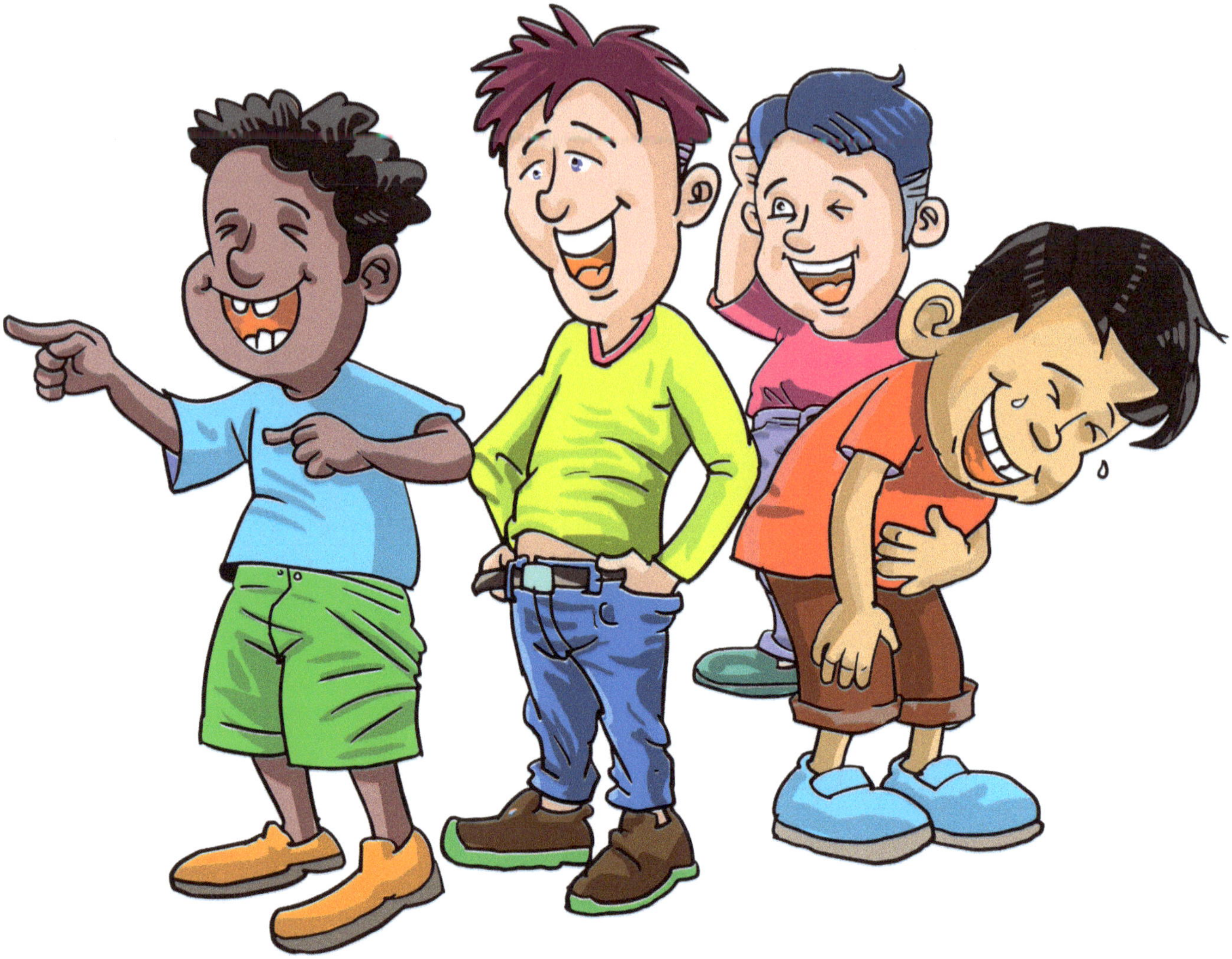

There has to be an audience for a belch.
If there's no one there, it's just a burp.

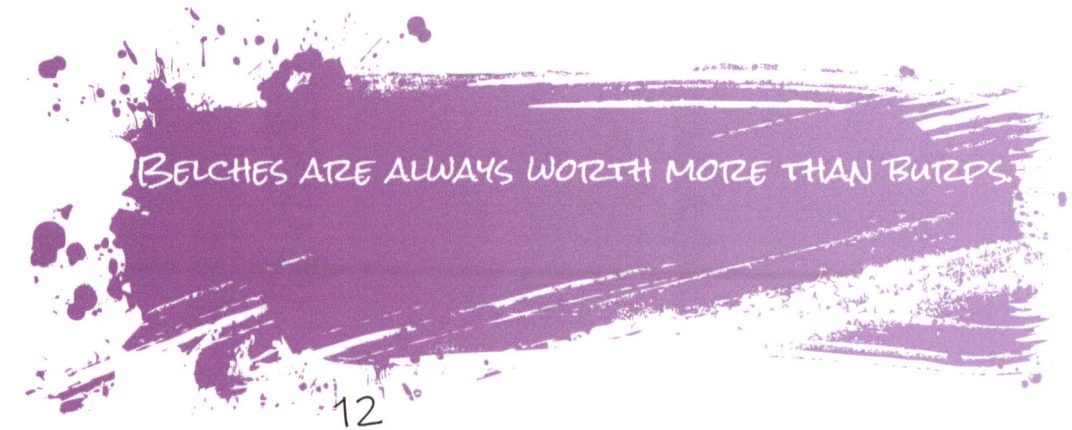
BELCHES ARE ALWAYS WORTH MORE THAN BURPS.

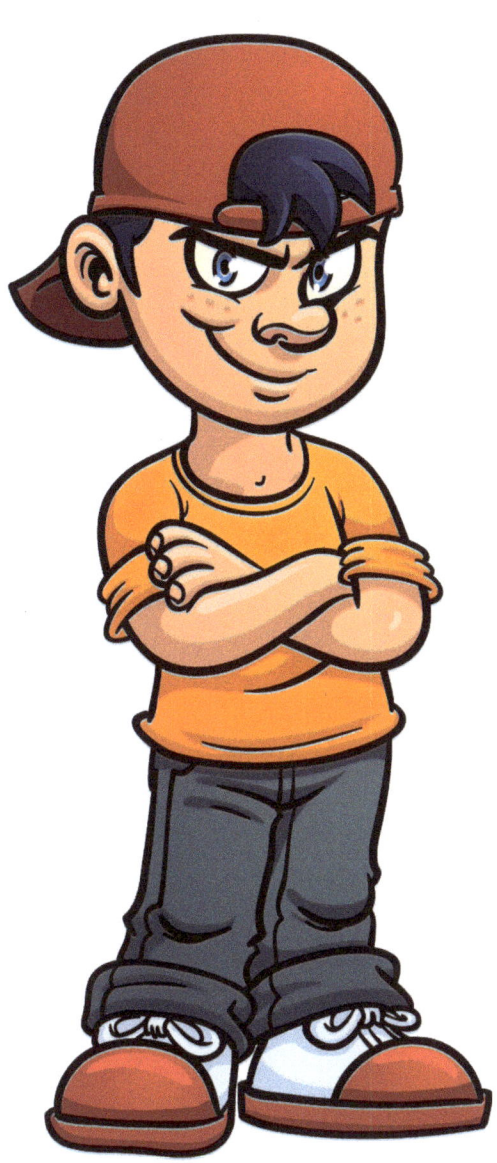

The audience might be your best friend, who thinks it's hilarious.

A BEST FRIEND BELCH IS WORTH 100 POINTS.

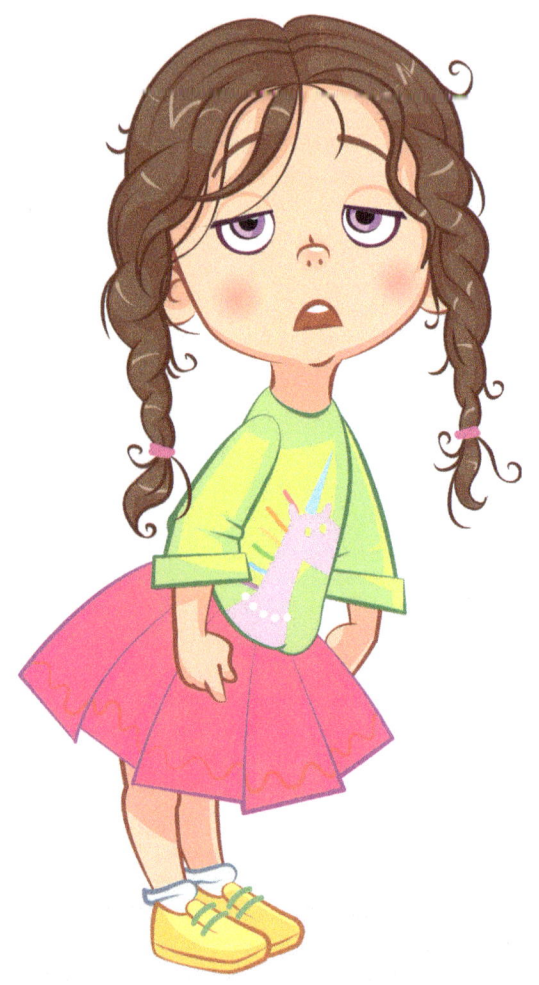

Or, it can be a girl (just about any girl), who thinks you're truly gross.

That means that girls are worth 200 points. (If you are a girl, you get 1000 points just for reading this book.) And girls get double points on every page.

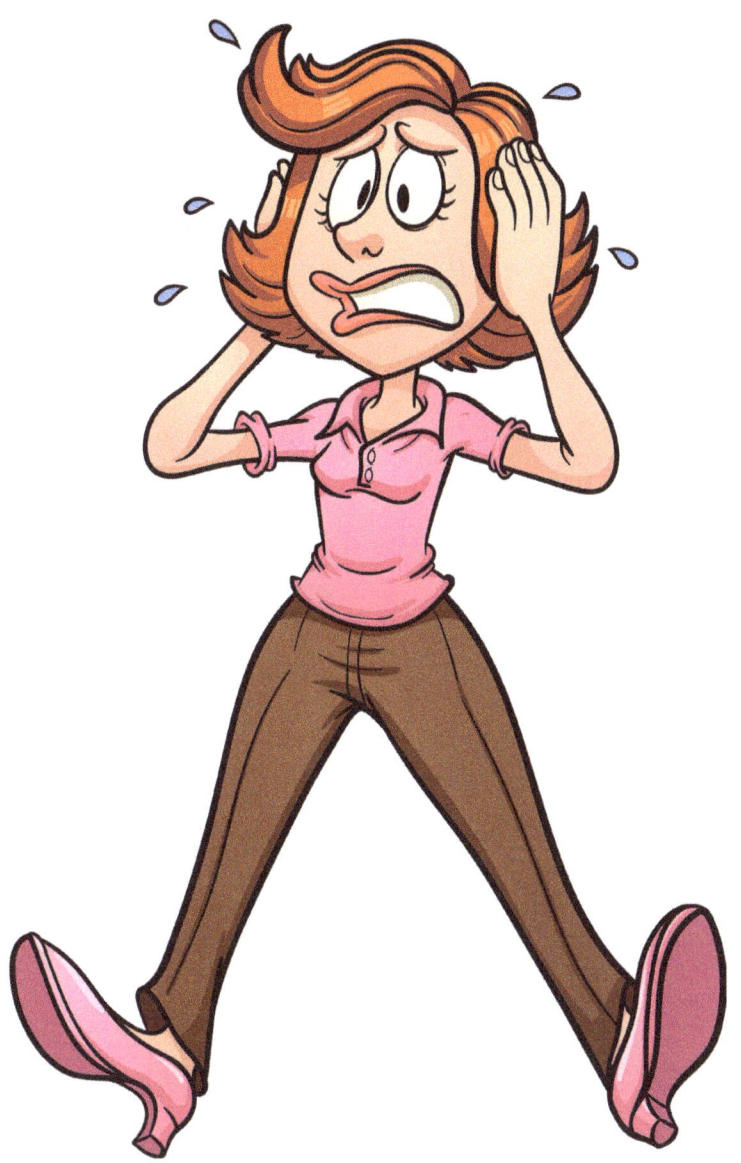

It can be your mom, who thinks it's horrible that you think it's so funny.

Moms are too easy, so she's only worth 50 points.

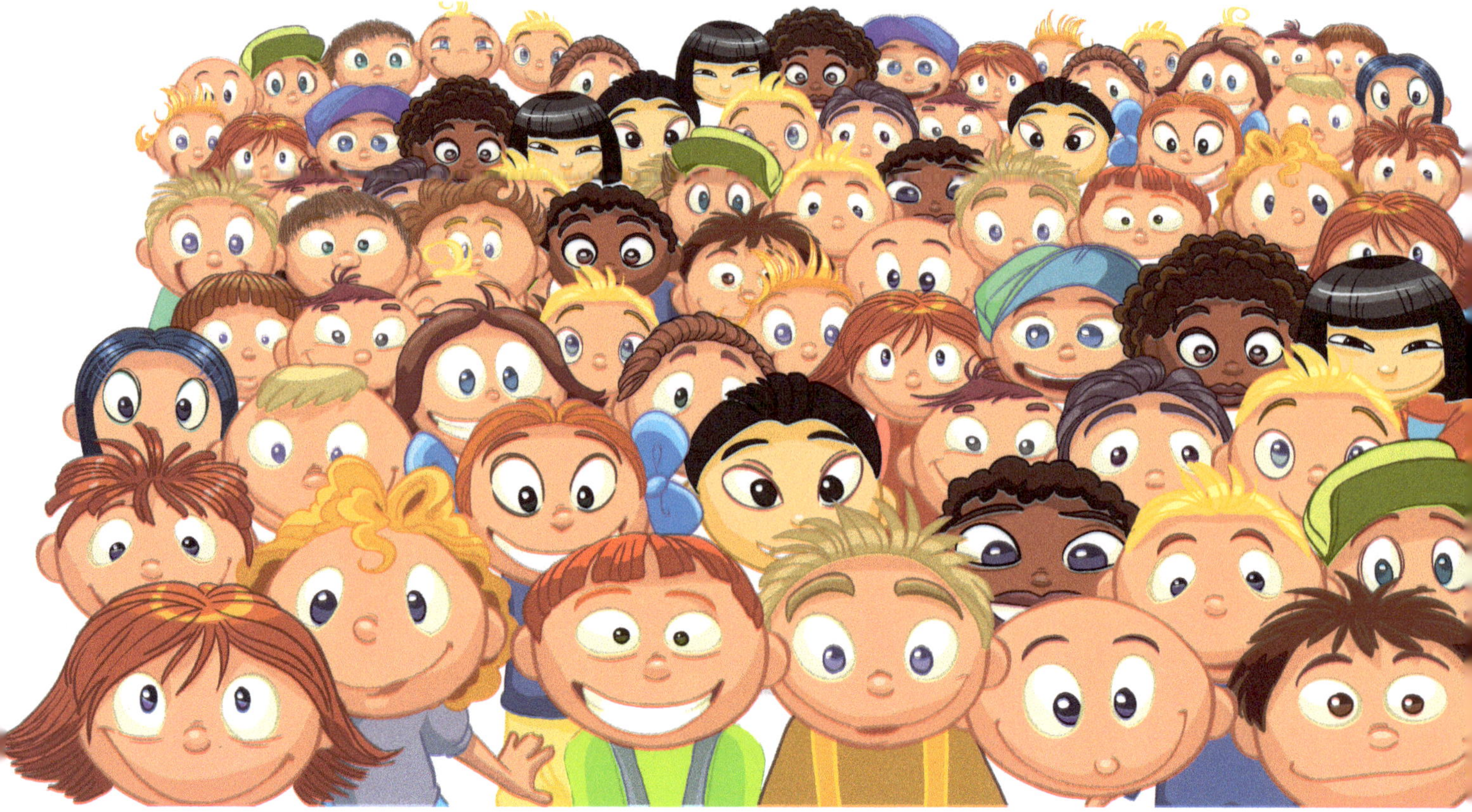

Or your entire class.

That means there will be a teacher (who disapproves) but can't do much about it.

(Even better, a Sunday School teacher, minister, rabbi, or other clergy.)

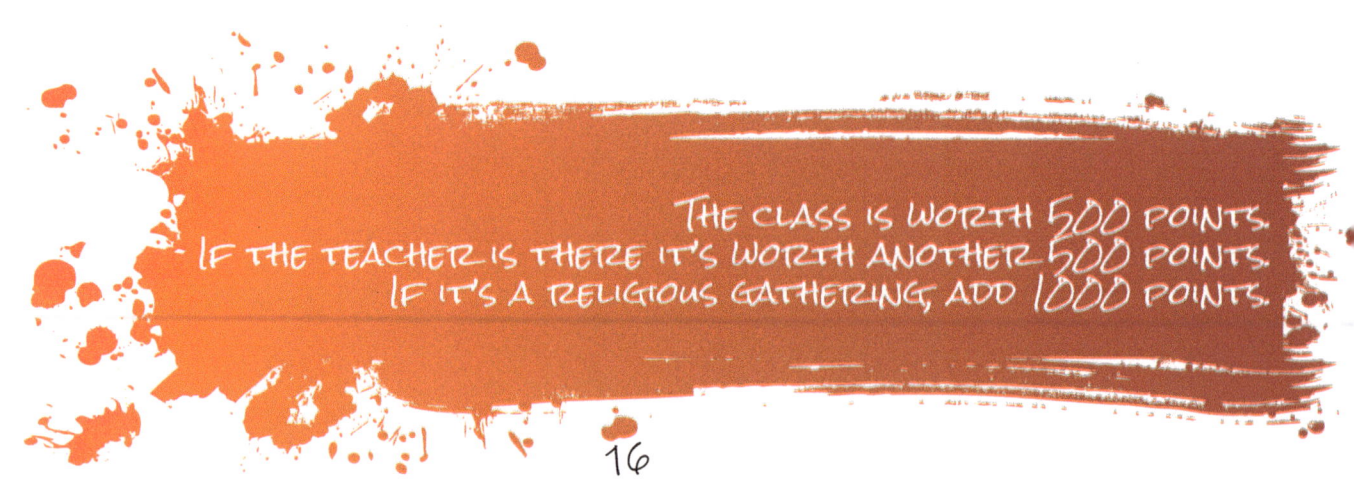

The class is worth 500 points.
If the teacher is there it's worth another 500 points.
If it's a religious gathering, add 1000 points.

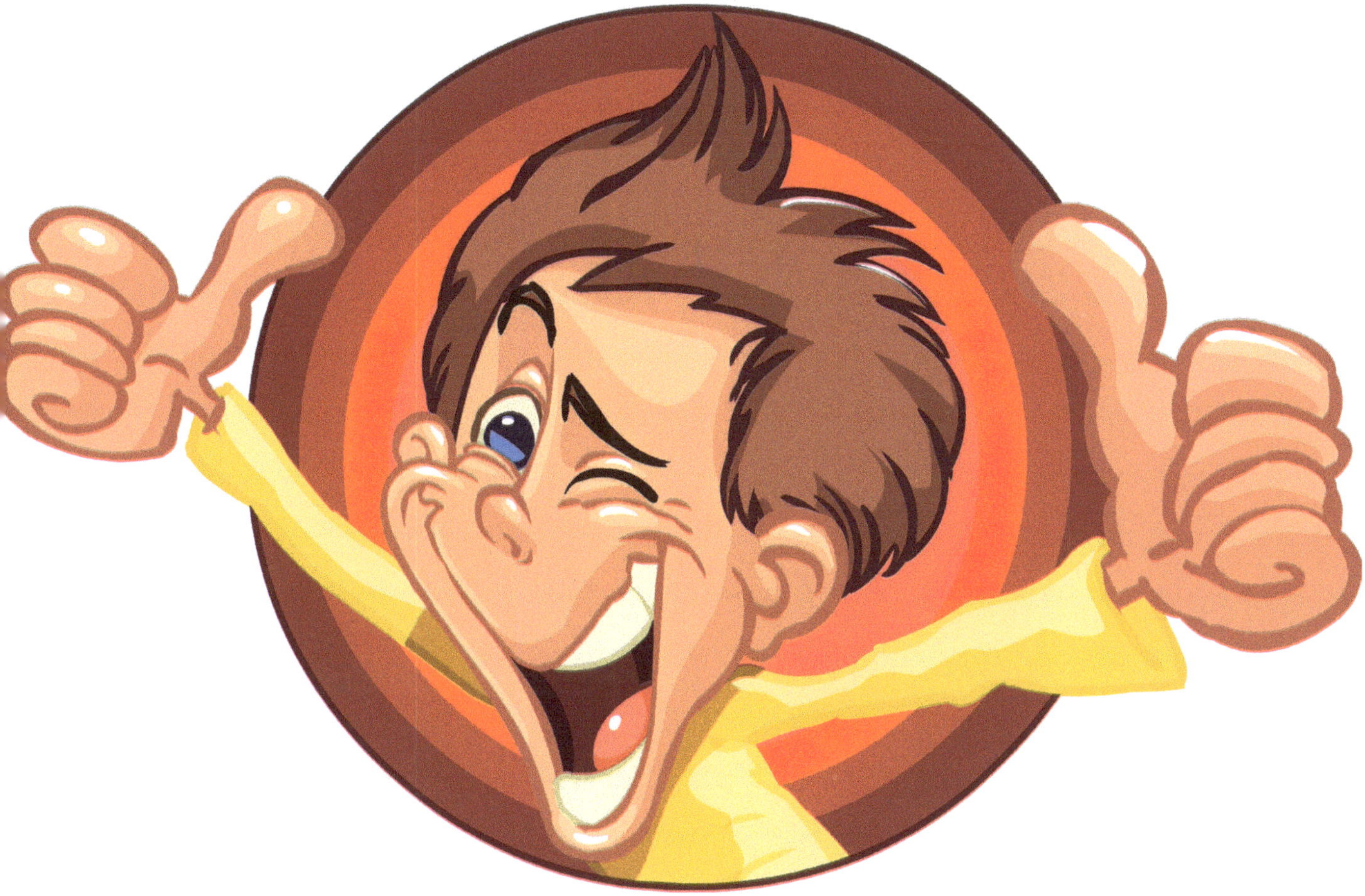

The reason you burp and belch is usually that something you've eaten is being digested, which can produce gas that climbs your throat and comes out your mouth.

Face it, belches are mouth farts. And that means they're funny.

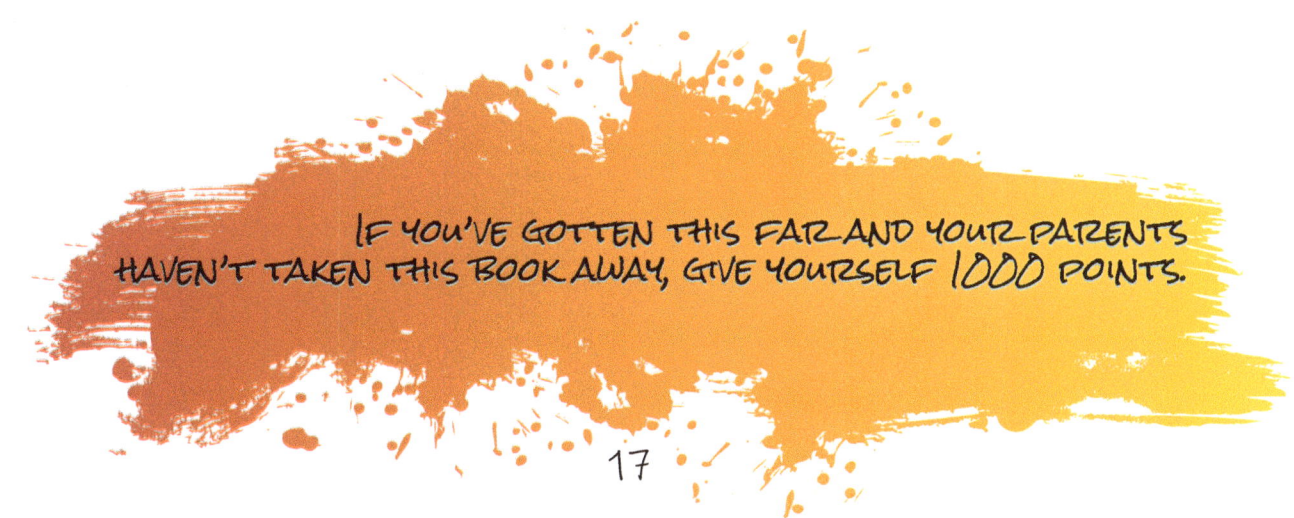

IF YOU'VE GOTTEN THIS FAR AND YOUR PARENTS HAVEN'T TAKEN THIS BOOK AWAY, GIVE YOURSELF 1000 POINTS.

THE END

Unless you want to read about vomit.

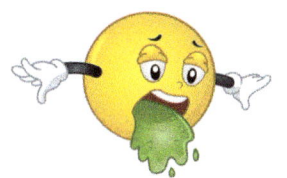

PART III
BARFING

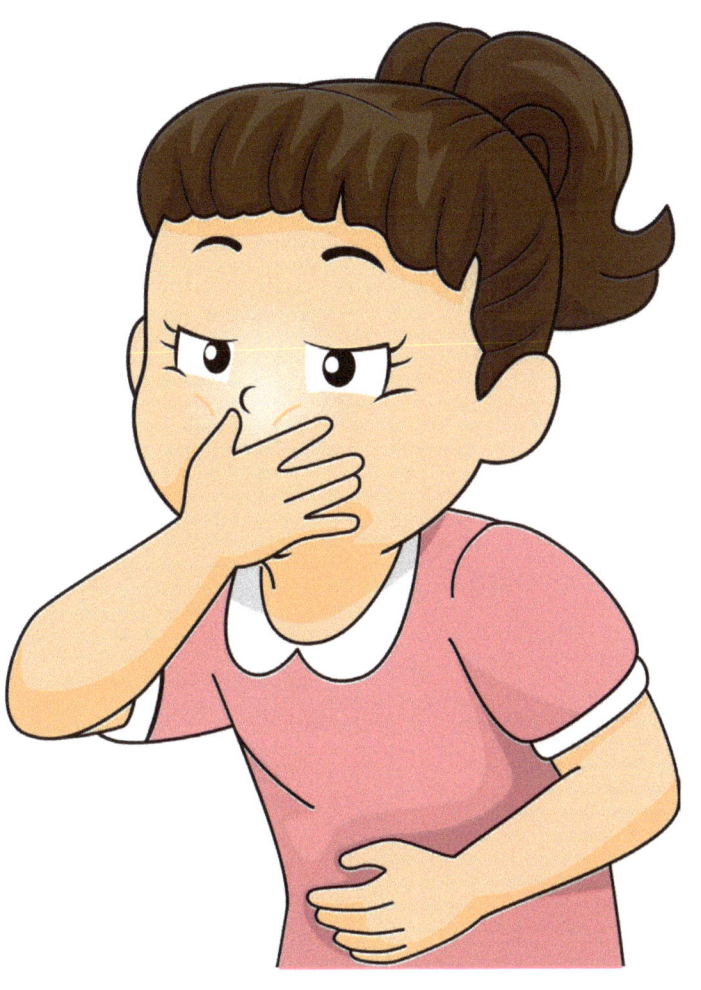

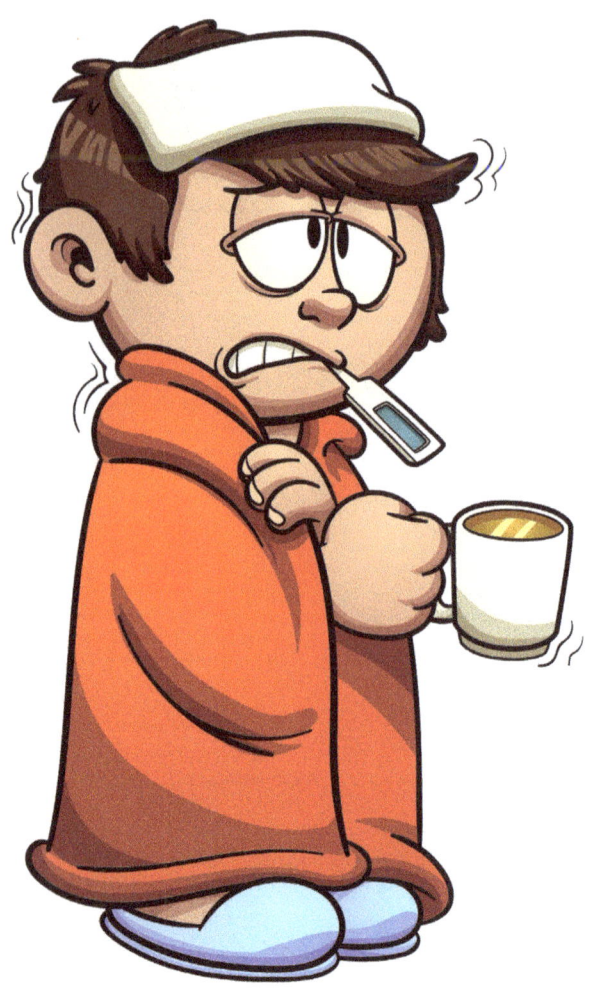

It usually happens when you're not feeling well. You may be really sick or you may just be feeling uneasy for some reason.

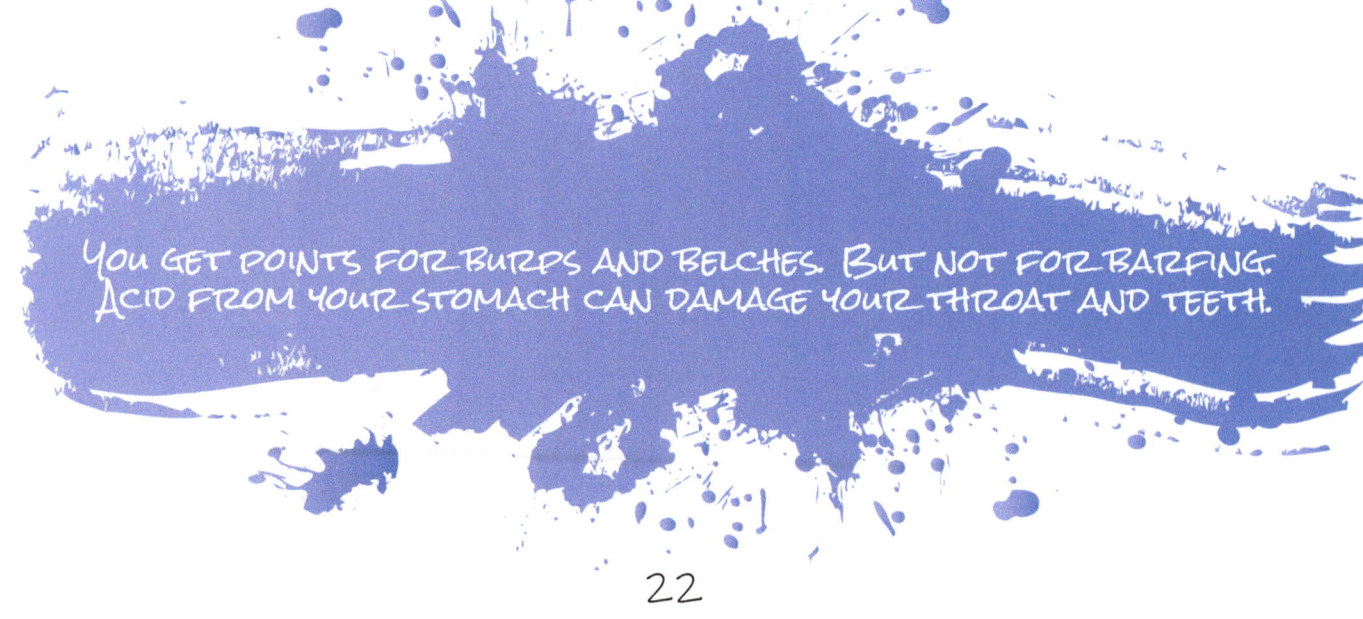

You get points for burps and belches. But not for barfing. Acid from your stomach can damage your throat and teeth.

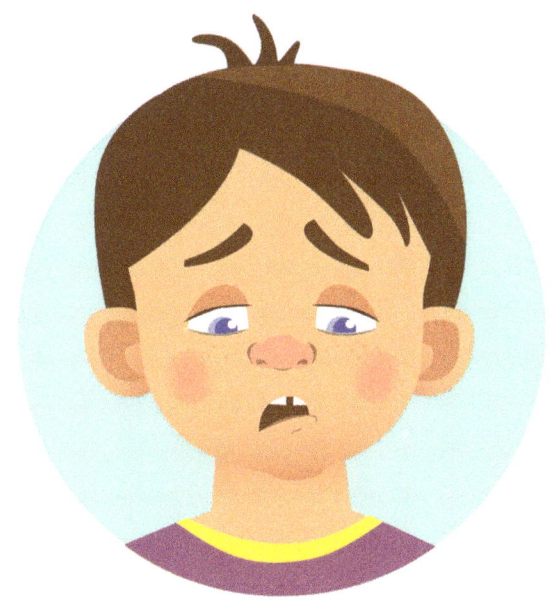

Barfing is not funny – not to the person barfing – until much, much later.

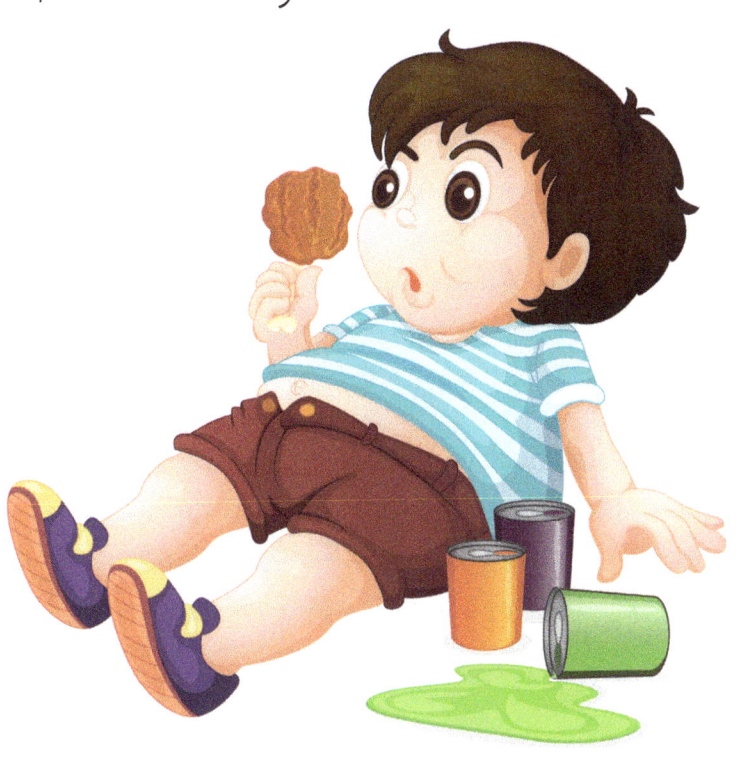

But when you're barfing, it can be hilarious to your friends, especially if you brought it on yourself by eating or drinking too much. (Feeling "crapulous" means you've been overeating.)

No points. No points at all.

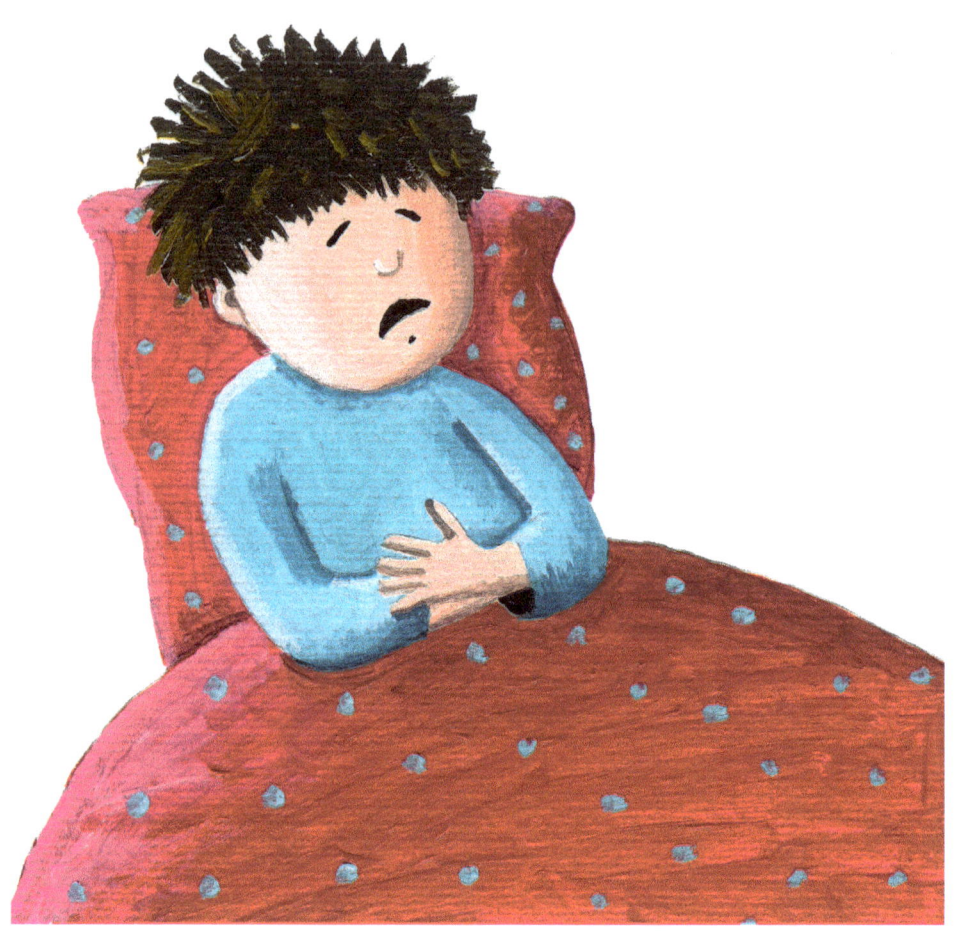

There's that uneasy period before it happens, when you know it's coming.

There are names for that unhappy time: nausea, queasiness, biliousness, squeamishness, gagging, gurping, and sometimes boke.

It could be that you're sick or have an upset stomach, but it could be something else.

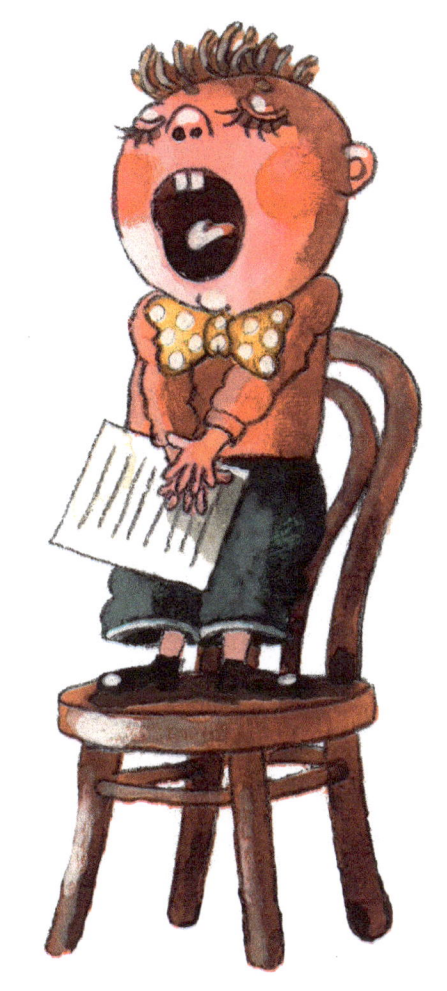

Maybe you've got a stressful event happening – a test, a speech, a recital, or a wedding that you're in.

But you can feel it coming, so you have to make a choice.

Do you mention it to someone and try to get help?

Or, do you try to tough it out?

Good luck...

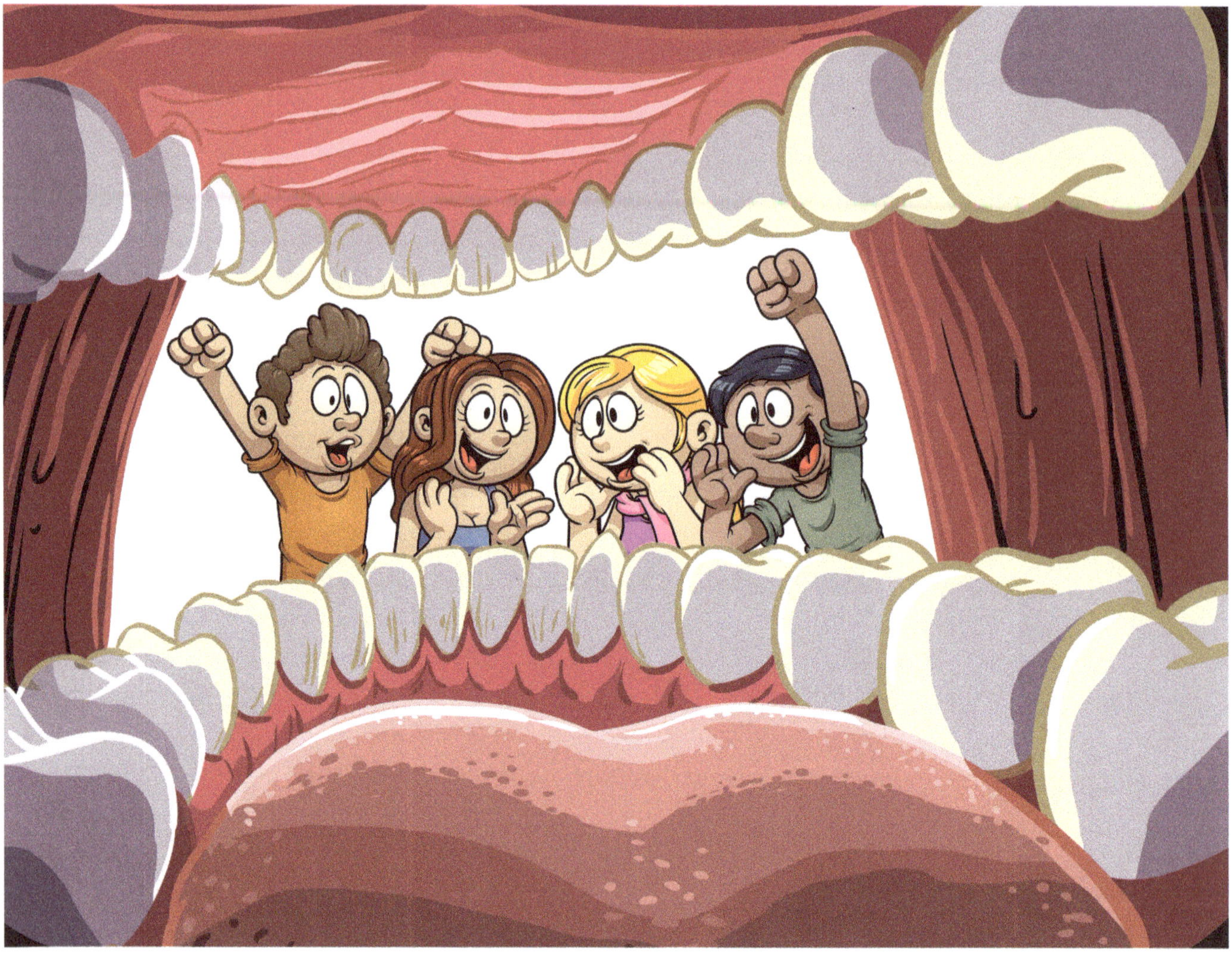

You don't want to make fun of someone who is barfing — unless they do it themselves.

Or — at least wait until they feel better.

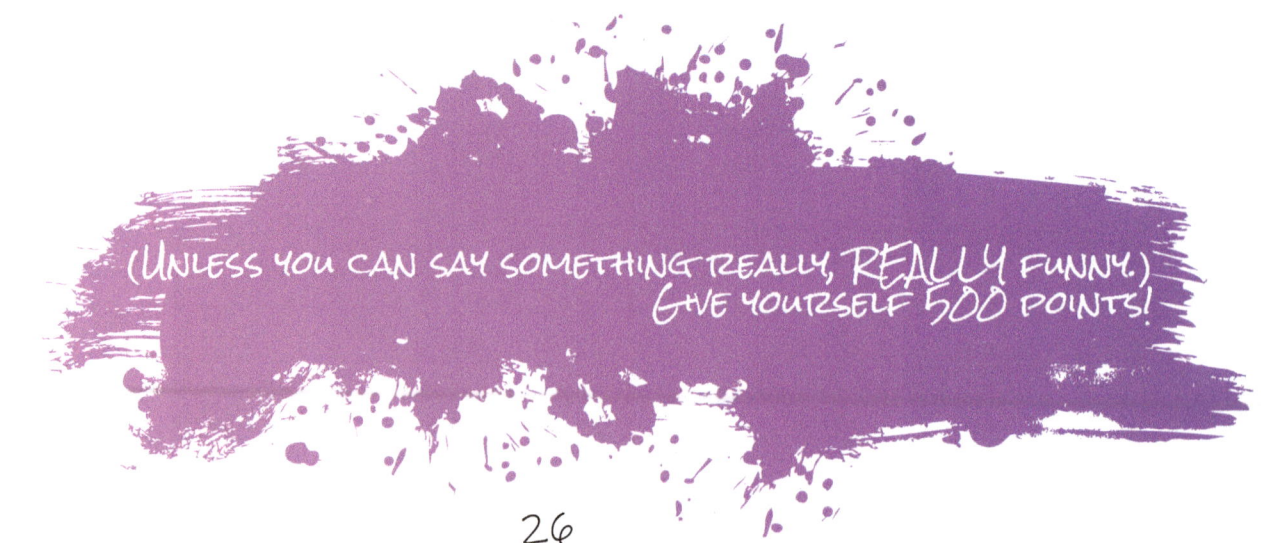
(UNLESS YOU CAN SAY SOMETHING REALLY, REALLY FUNNY.) GIVE YOURSELF 500 POINTS!

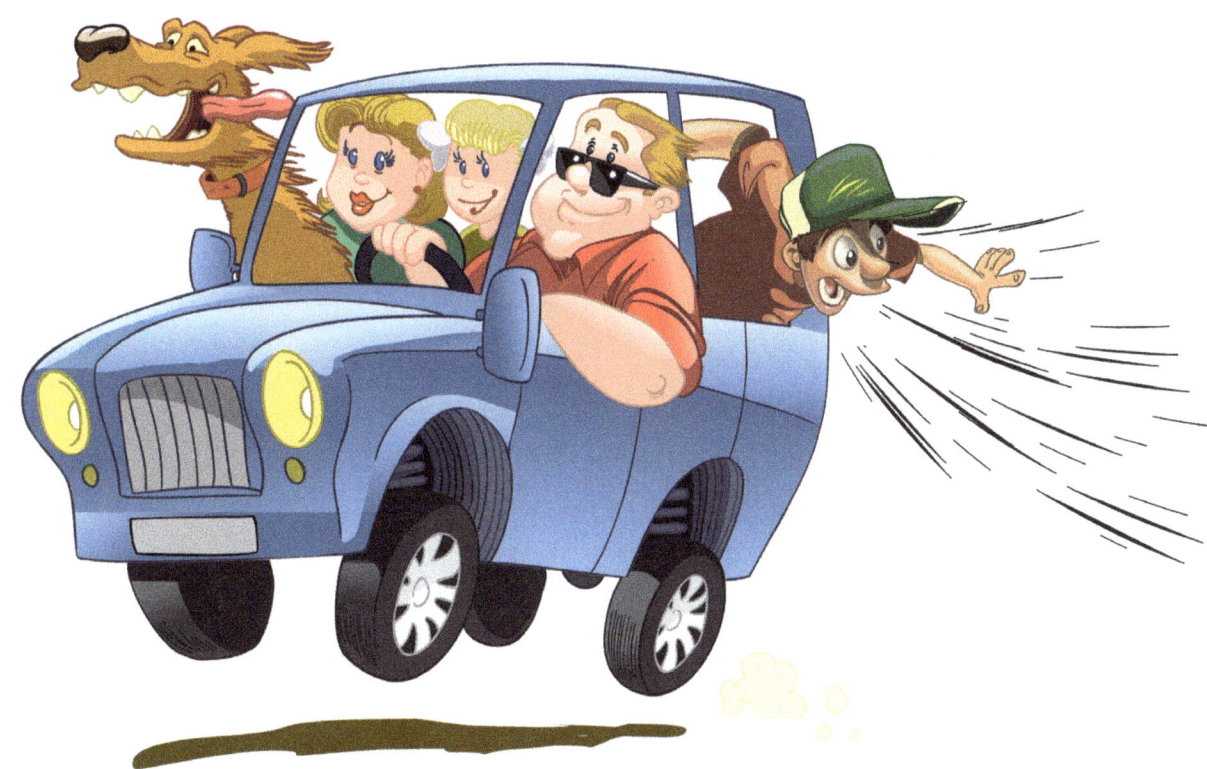

Motion sickness can do it.

Perhaps you're "carsick." The proper word for that is "kinesia" or "kinetosis" – but if you use these words, don't expect anyone to understand that you want them to pull the car over.

It's terrible that a really great place for barfing is also one of the worst places – your parents' car. The good news is that there's a window you can open.

But – if you don't wait for your parents to pull over and stop, whatever you spew out the window is going to blow right back into your face.

Double-yuk!!!

THAT'S WORTH A LOT OF POINTS. AS MANY POINTS AS YOU WANT!

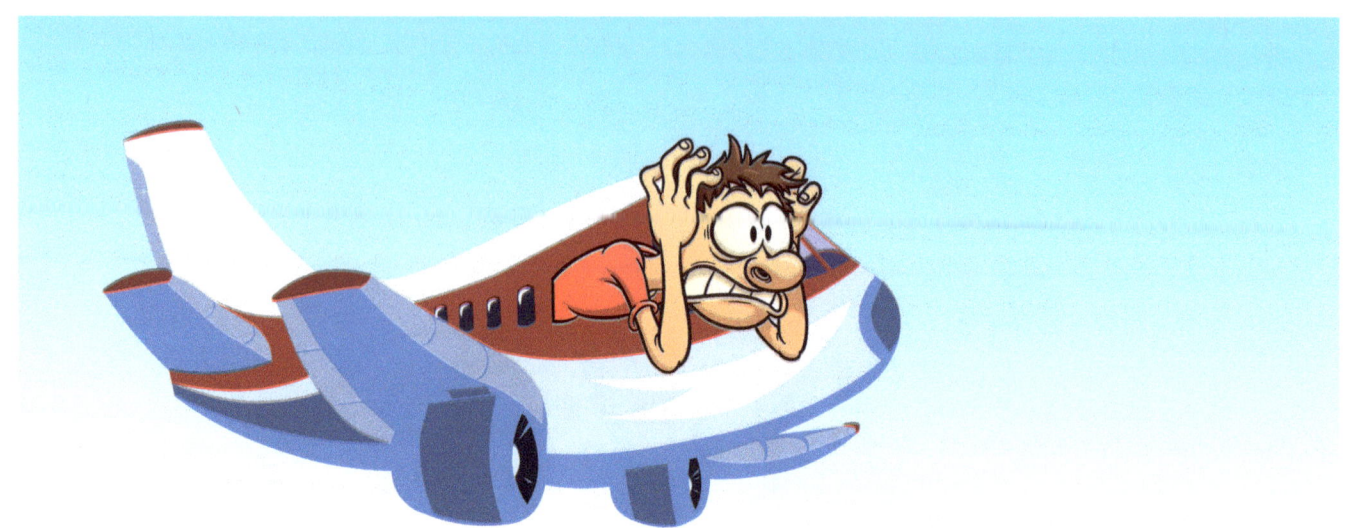

If you're on an airplane you could be "airsick," but you definitely know that no one's going to pull over for you. Luckily, airplane seats have little paper bags for that. And they're free!

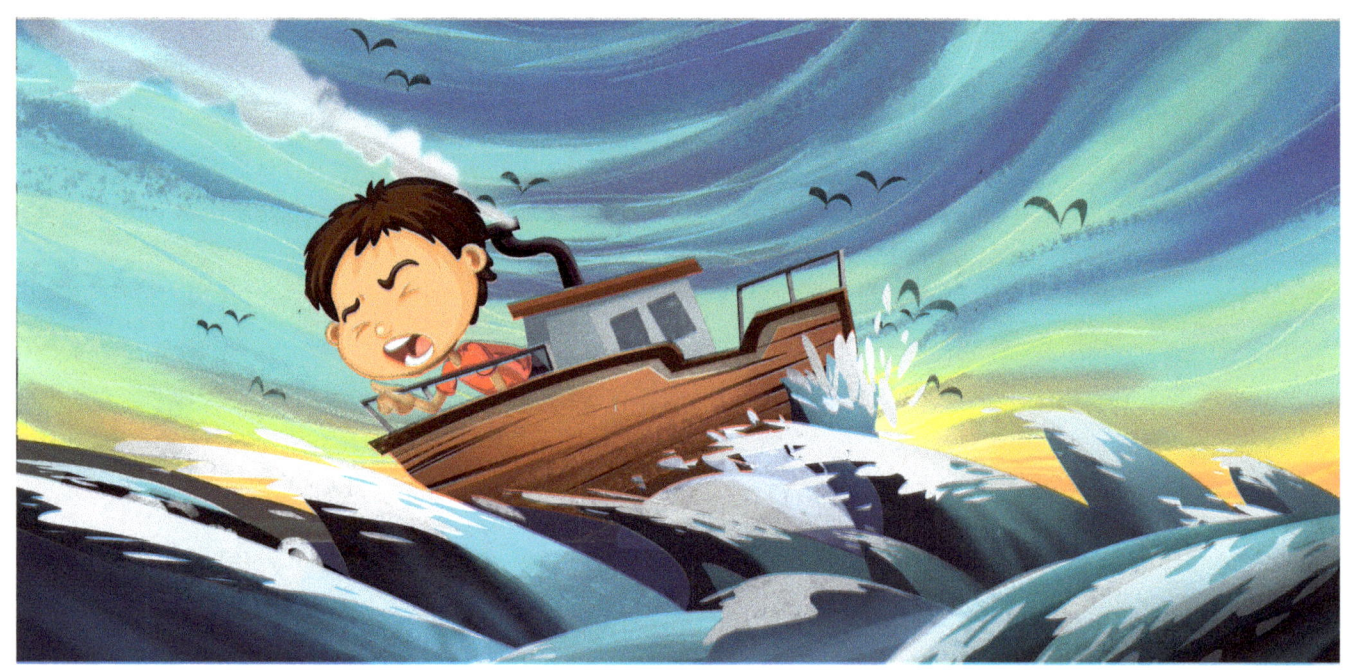

Boats can make you "seasick," but they don't need to pull over. Just stick your head over the railing and let go. That's called "chumming." You may hear the French term, which is "mal de mer."

And, there's something called "morning sickness." Ask your mom about that.

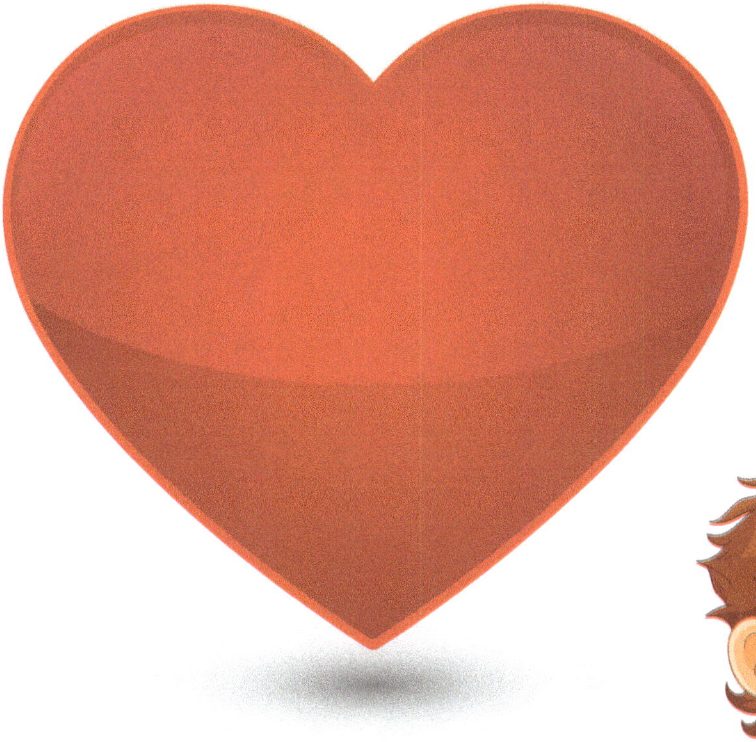

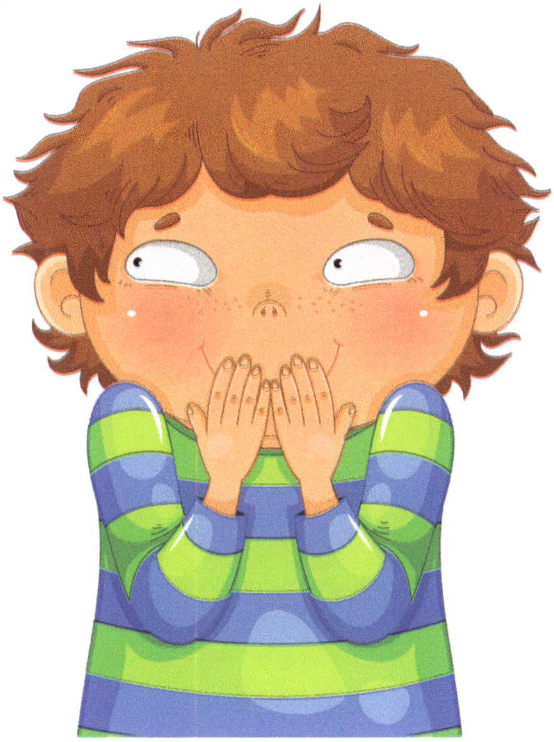

Being "lovesick" can do it, too.

In a weird way it's somehow considered romantic that love can make you throw up.

(But if you do barf, it's not romantic at all.)

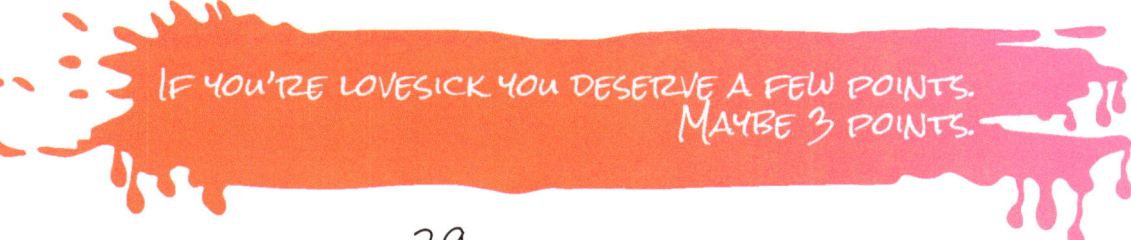
IF YOU'RE LOVESICK YOU DESERVE A FEW POINTS. MAYBE 3 POINTS.

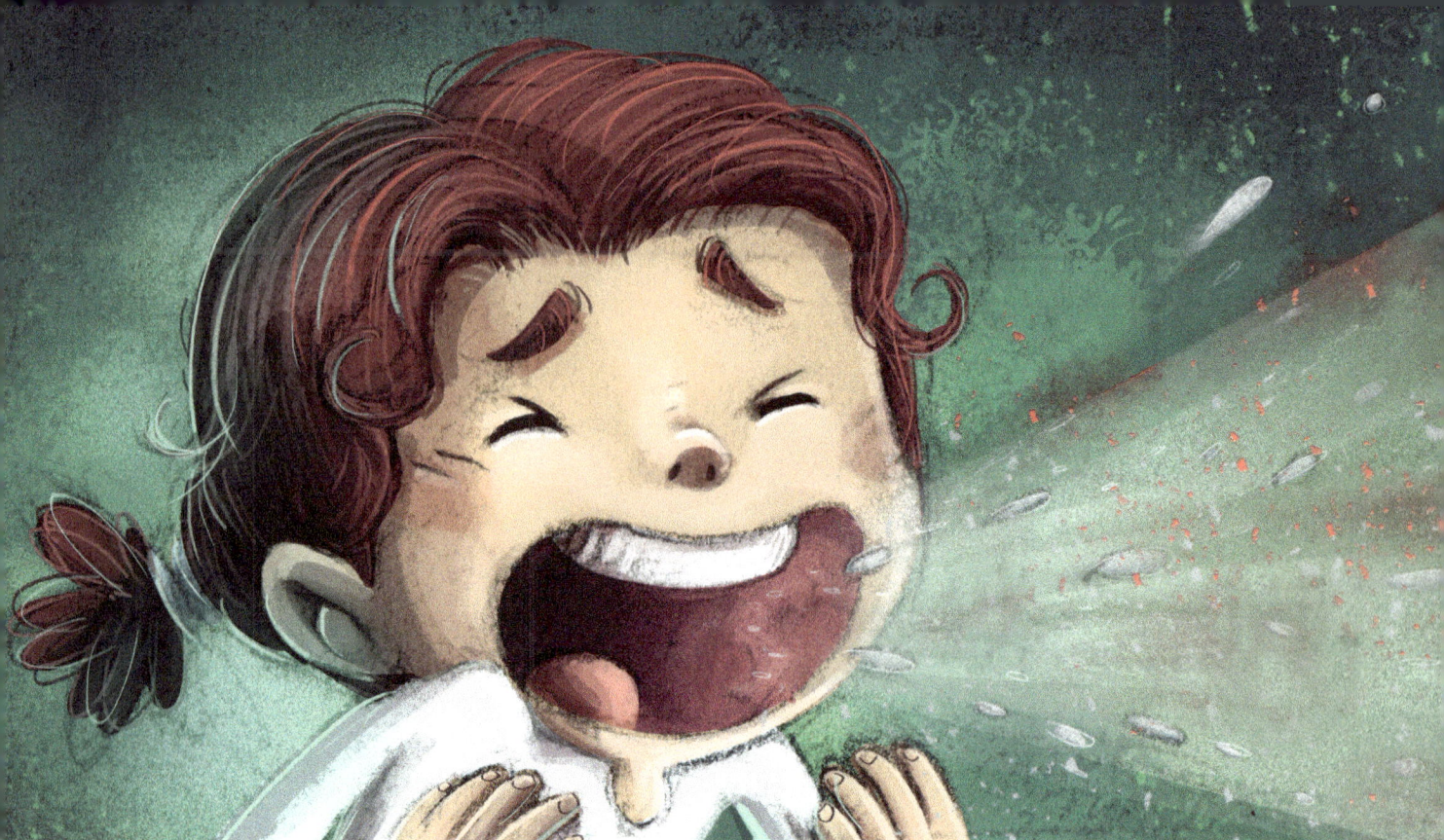

Barfing can be violent and uncontrollable, or reluctant and gradual, and sometimes it can even take coaxing.

There may come a time when you need to throw up — you may even want to throw up — but for some reason nothing comes out. Maybe you haven't eaten for a while, or maybe you've already thrown up everything you've got.

When you keep trying, you can get the "dry heaves." It's no fun and you go through all the unpleasantness of being sick for no real result. Some people call that "burking."

Sometimes when you barf, you just get a little dribble of drool. Other times, unfortunately, stuff comes flying out in a primordial form of target practice called "projectile vomiting."

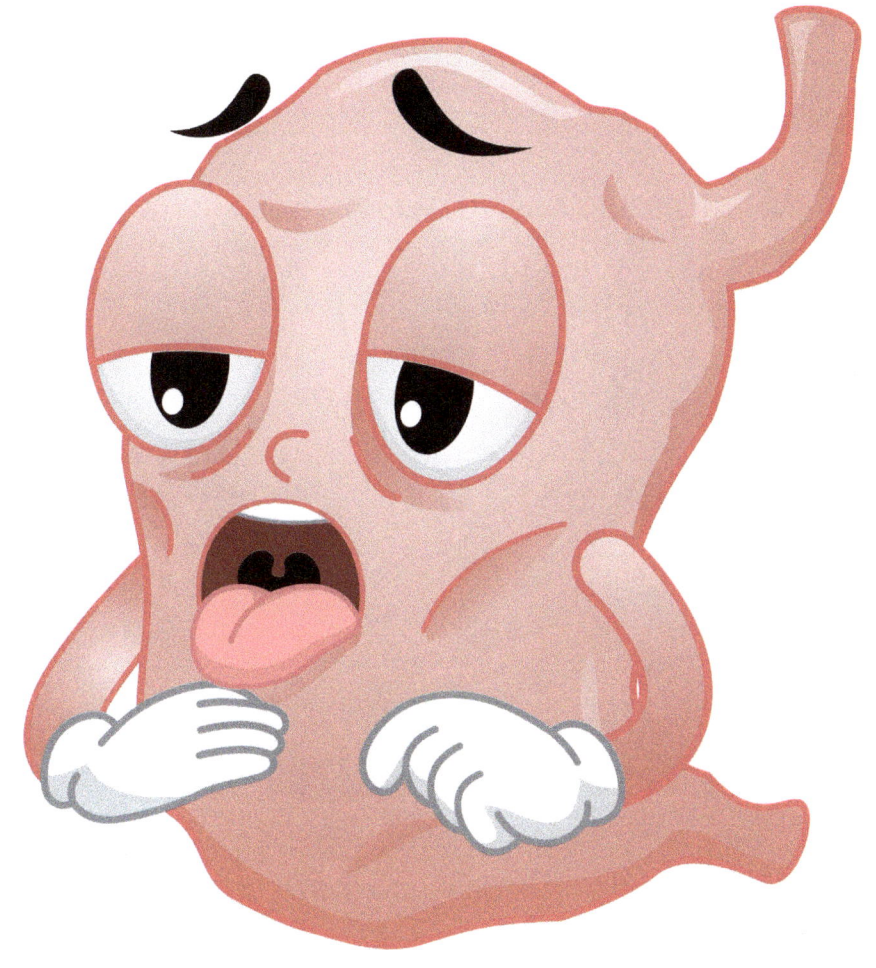

Basically, the usual reason you barf is that there is something awful inside your body that shouldn't be there. (That's why it's so disgusting.) And it wants out, one way or another.

If you were full of songs and rainbows there wouldn't be a problem.

Bad fish? Big problem. Too much cake and ice cream? Better call Ralph.

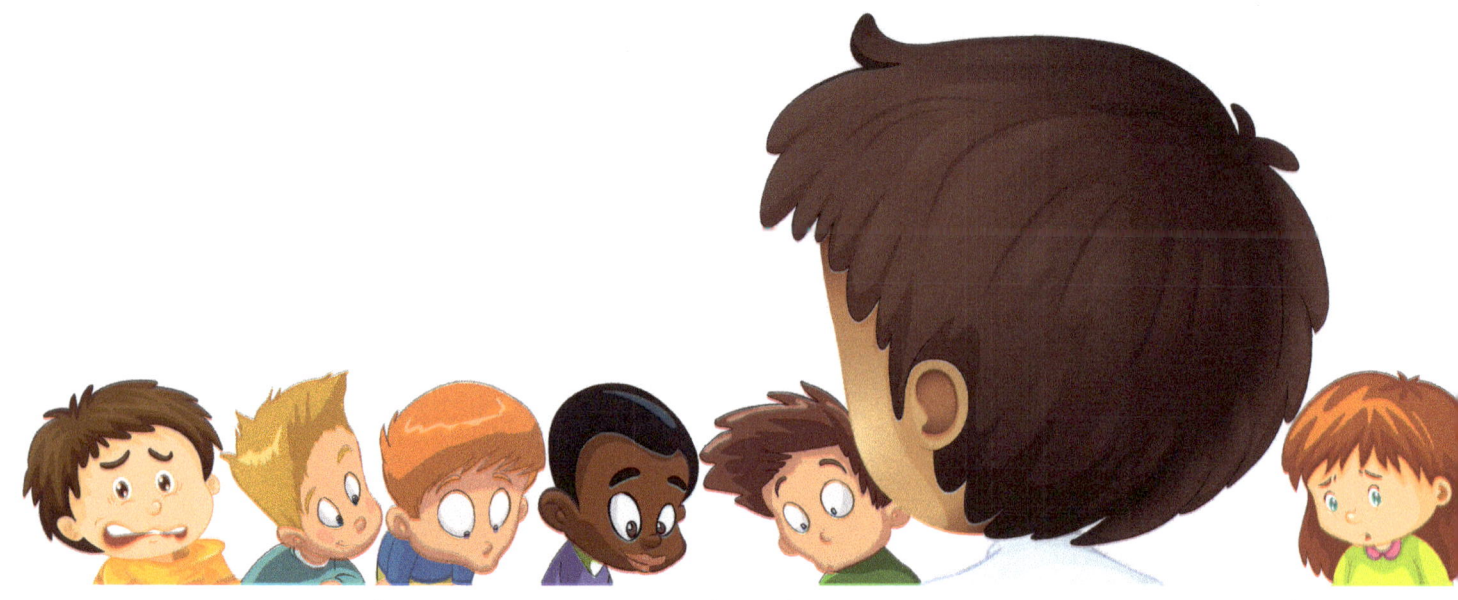

For some people, seeing someone barf is enough to make them do the same. That's just one of the fun things about barfing. It's hilariously contagious.

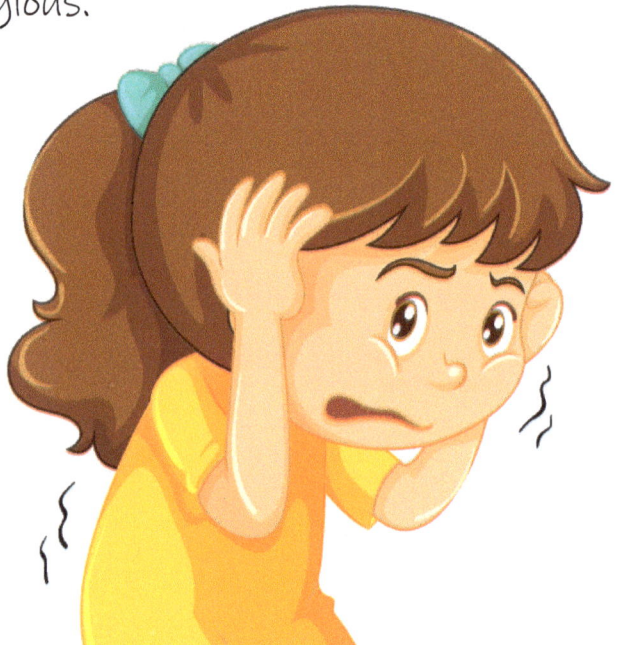

Sometimes just hearing the word "vomit" (or whatever word you use) is enough to make someone barf.

Not that you should try, but if it "happens" give yourself 500 points.

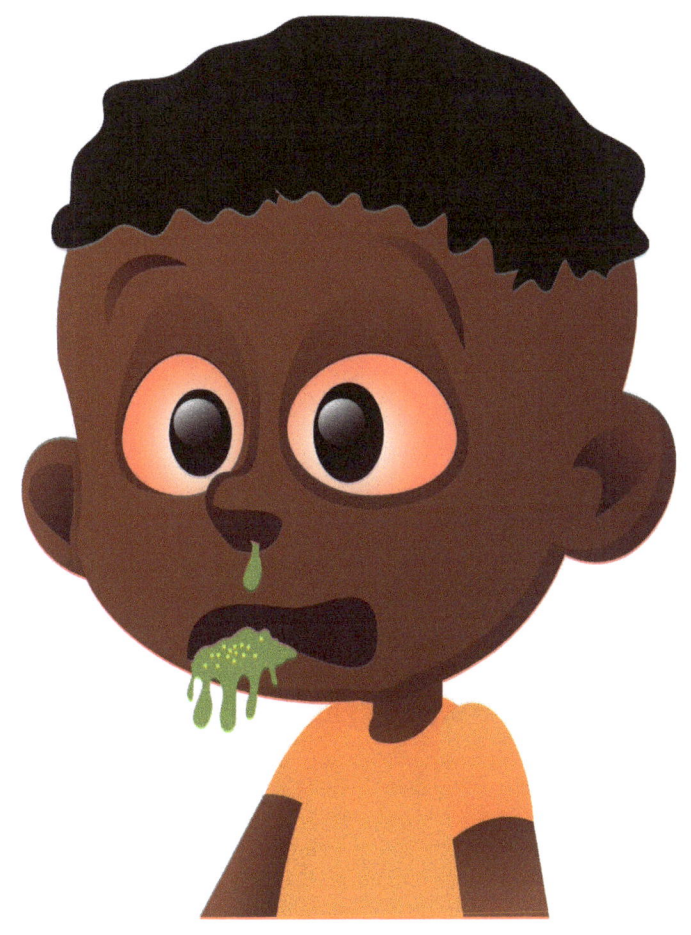

If you're eating and someone unexpectedly makes you laugh really hard, sometimes food comes out of your mouth and nose. That's called "snarfing."

IF YOU SAY SOMETHING SO FUNNY THAT YOUR BUDDY SNARFS, GIVE YOURSELF 100 POINTS.

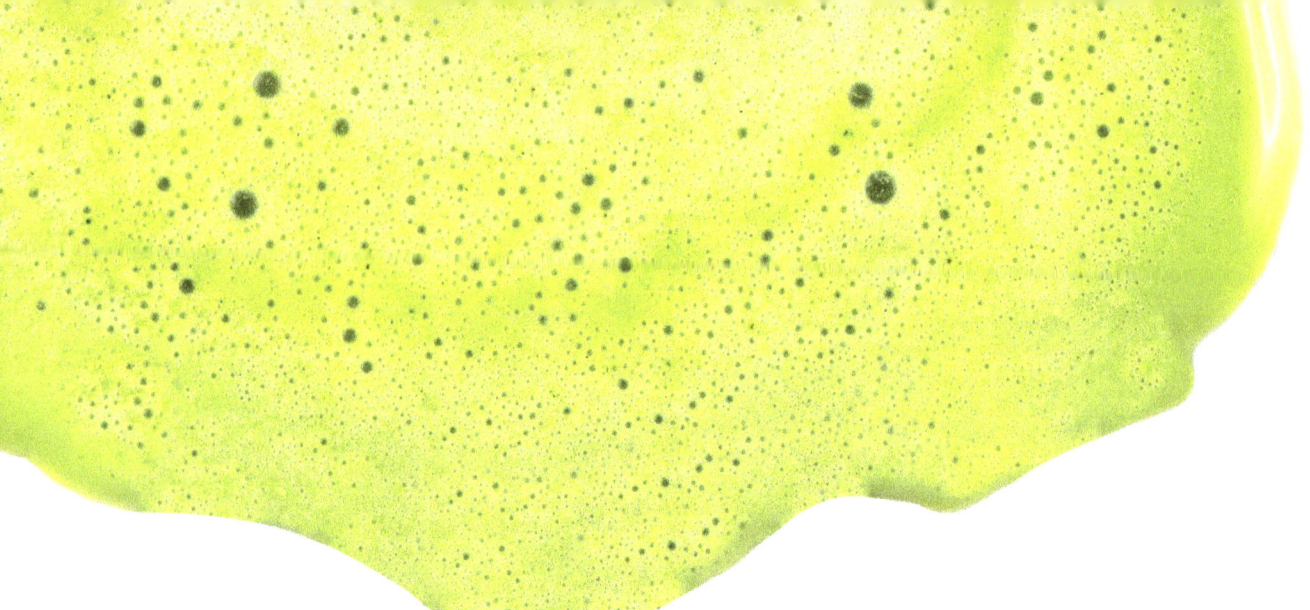

What's the best thing to call barf? What else can you say?

Let's face it. "Vomit" is kind of a clinical term and a little rude. "Spit up" seems childish and "throw up" is just boring.

Do you know a better word?

These are some common examples you may know:

Upchuck	Heave	Hurl
Spew	Unswallow	Regurgitate
Puke	Gag	Ralph

5 POINTS FOR NOT BARFING WHEN YOU READ THESE WORDS.

GLOSSARY

Here are a few choice words for barfing. Which one will you use when you talk to your doctor? Circle your favorites.

Yuke	York	Zork
Boff	Boot	Bolking
Emit	Uneat	Hiccup
Perk	Yack	Cack
Expel	Yak	Rucking
Gush	Gragg	Rifting
Disgorg	Bargle	Routing
Cast	Chorkle	Bring up
Cat	Shunder	Boking
Bob	Yarf	Perking
Posseting	Braf	Braking
Burl	Yatch	Groaning
Yarf	Quease	Suspiring
Fergle	Charfus	Grelk

25 POINTS FOR EVERY WORD YOU CIRCLED.

Because barfing has been around since the cavemen, there are lots of words for it. Some of them go way back. For instance, Shakespeare used "puke" back in 1600 in his play "As You Like It." (Hint: You won't like it.)

Rumor has it that some ancient Romans had a special room called a vomitorium just for barfing during feasts. It's not true, but it should be.

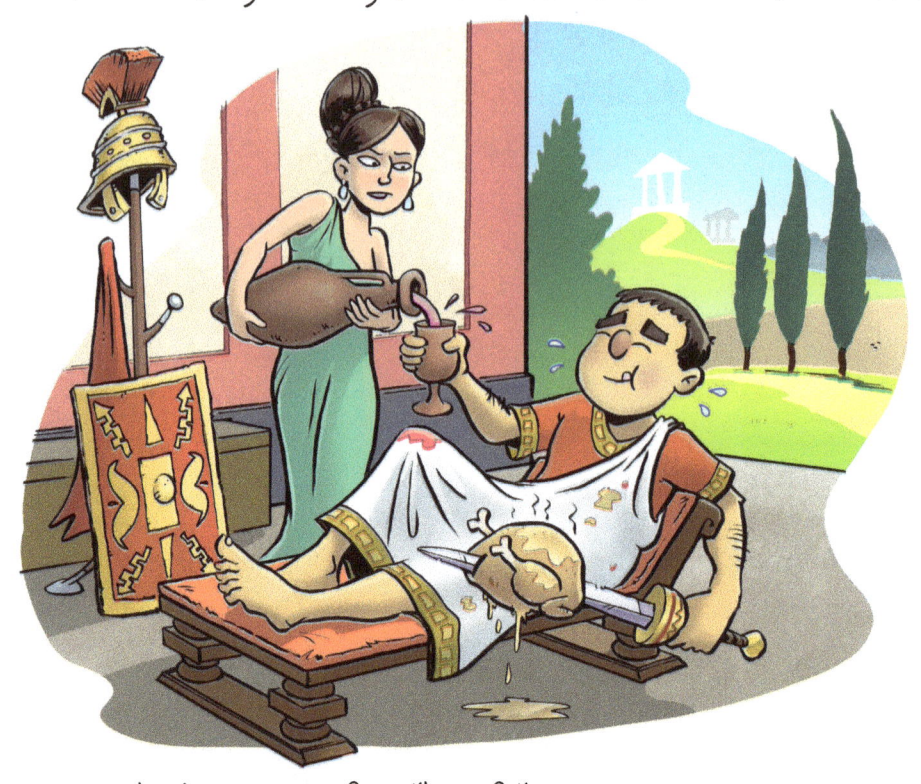

Here are some archaic terms for "barf."

Purge

Disembogue

Cascade

Regorge

Brake

Cascade

Parbreak

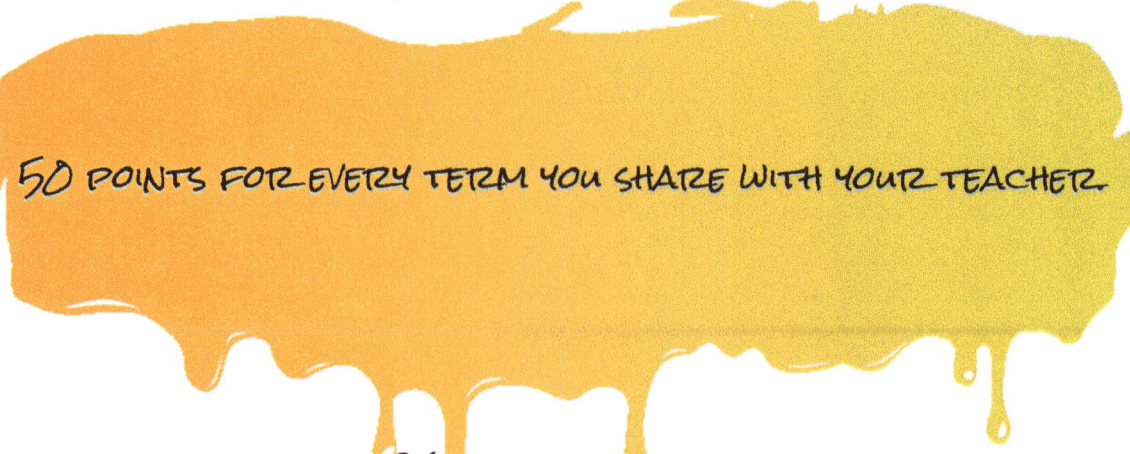

50 POINTS FOR EVERY TERM YOU SHARE WITH YOUR TEACHER

There are words for the act of barfing (verbs) and there are words for the result of barfing (nouns).

VERBS

When you are barfing, you are...

...honking
...yeeching
...kecking
...egurgitating
...yorping

...yodeling
...purging
...spurting
...grelking
...booting

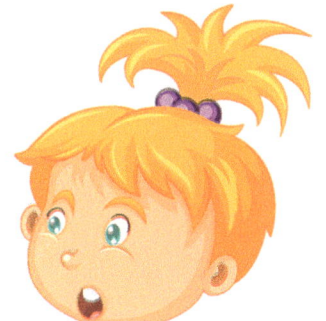

NOUNS

After barfing, you have a puddle of...

...vomitus
...parbreak
...pavement pizza
...liquid laugh
...effluvium

...ejectum
...the Technicolor yawn
...spue
...ejecta

"Barf" is one of those versatile words that can be both a verb and a noun. Likewise, when you "vomit" you bring up "vomit." You can "puke" "puke," too.

Here are other names that can be used both as a noun and as a verb:

Retch
Yark
Ulti

Chunder
Horf
Yoach

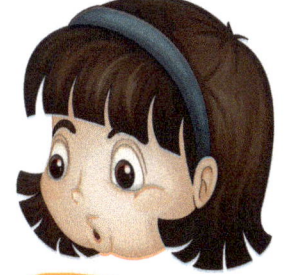

50 POINTS FOR EVERY WORD YOU USE BOTH WAYS IN A SENTENCE. IF IT GETS YOU IN TROUBLE, GIVE YOURSELF ANOTHER 500 POINTS.

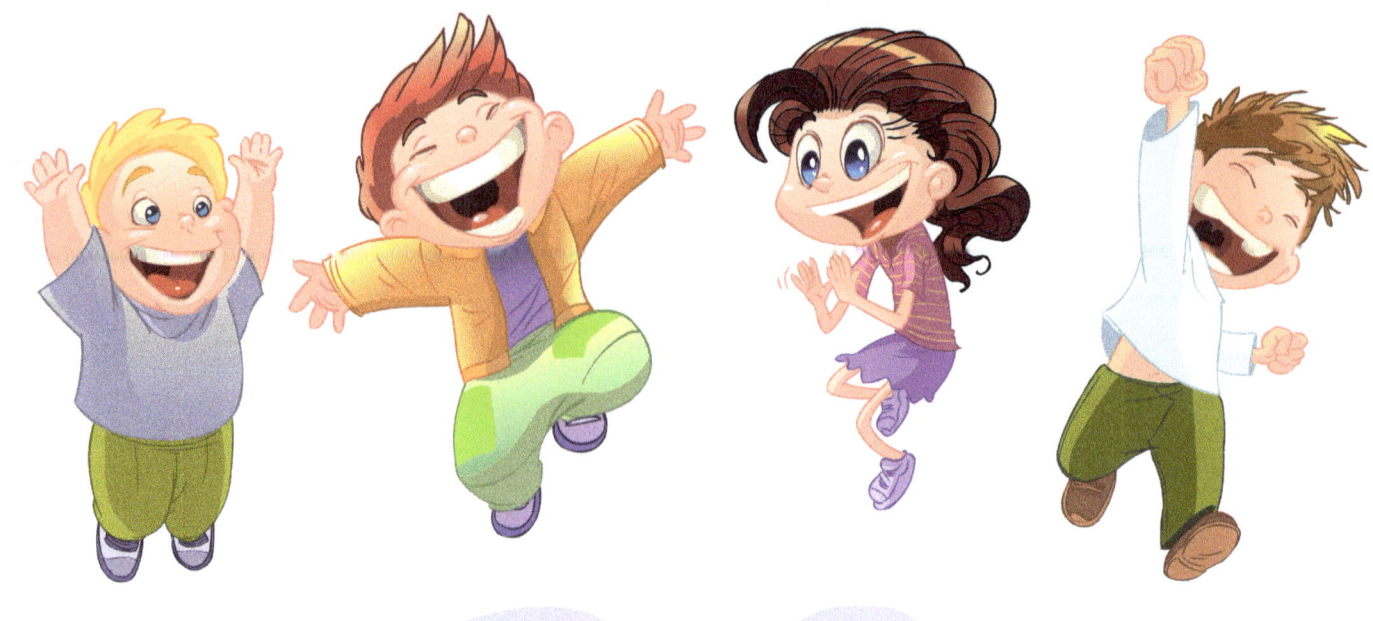

Many of the most descriptive words for "barf" come from the tortured sounds that people make as they do it.

Yell these words and see what it makes you think of. Stretch them out for the full effect.

Ralph or Raaaaaaaaallllllllppppphhhhh!!!

Retch or rettttttttccccccchhhhhhh!!!!

Urp or uuuuurrrrrrrrpppppppp!!!

Ughp or uggggggghhhhhpppppp!!!!

Brack or brrrrrrraaaaaaaaccccccckkkkkk!!!!

Urch or uuuuuurrrrrrrrccccccchhhhhhh!!!

Yoach or yooooooooaaaaaaaaccccccchhhhh!!!!

Hork or hhhhooooorrrrrrkkkkkk!!!

Blek or bbbblllleeeeeeeeeccccckkkkk!!!!

Yell them again REALLY loud for 100 points each. If it makes someone think you're sick, give yourself 500 points. If your yell makes someone actually barf, that's worth 1000 points.

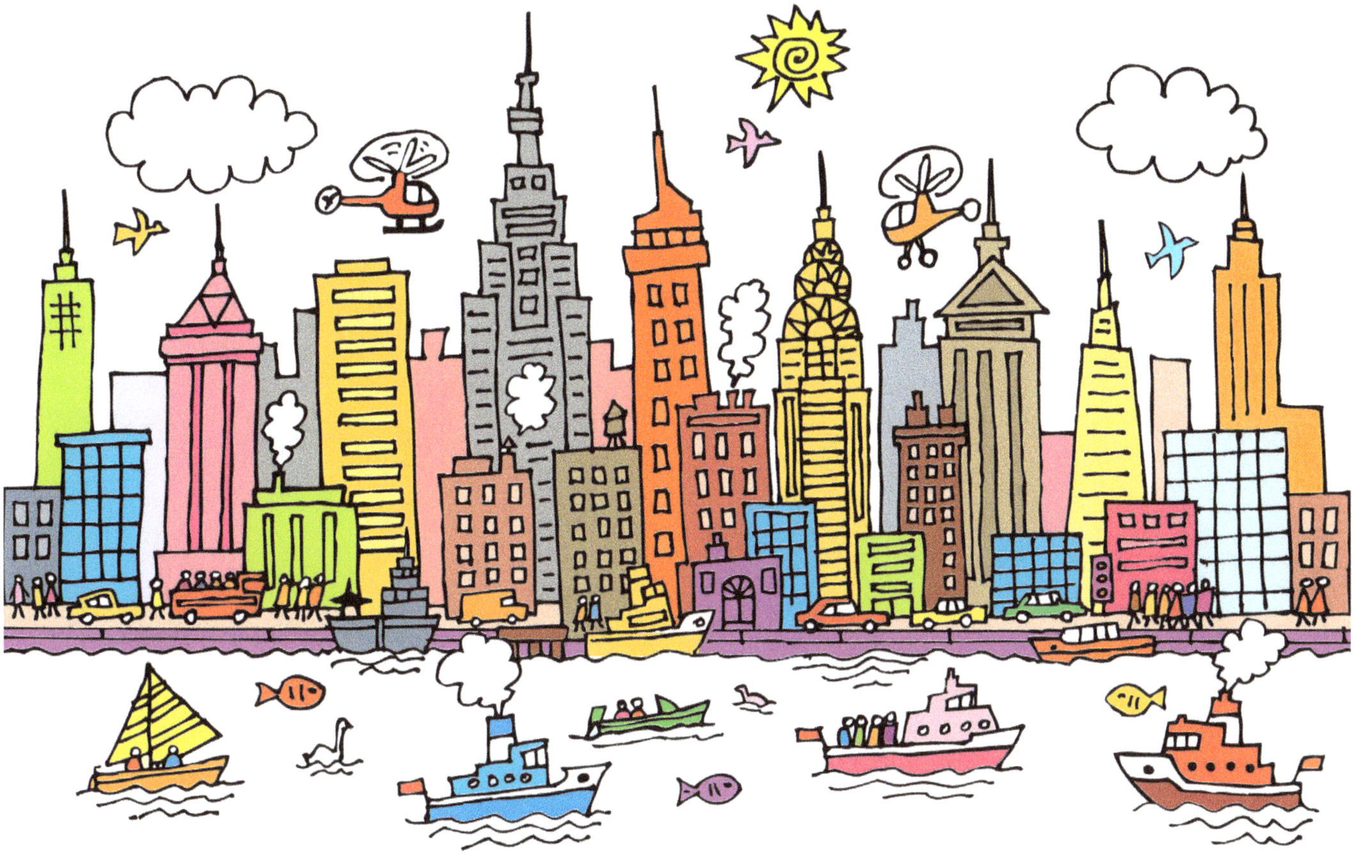

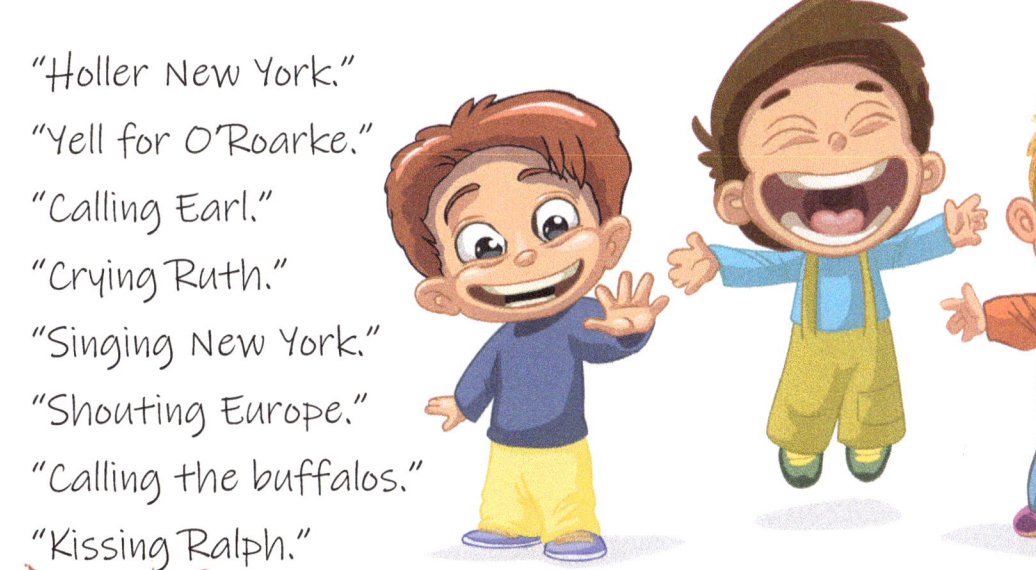

And there are expressions for barfing that are based on the sounds people make. Try them out.

"Holler New York."
"Yell for O'Roarke."
"Calling Earl."
"Crying Ruth."
"Singing New York."
"Shouting Europe."
"Calling the buffalos."
"Kissing Ralph."

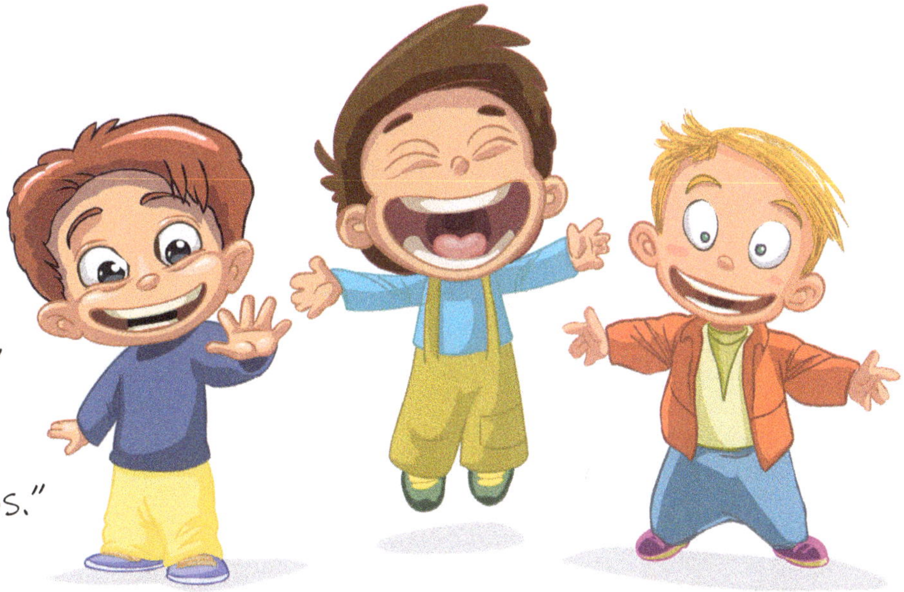

IF YOU CAN YELL (OR SING) THESE WORDS AND MAKE YOURSELF SOUND SICK, GIVE YOURSELF 1000 POINTS.

There are many colorful expressions for barfing, both disgusting and delightful. Some describe the act and some describe the awful product.

Having a spit.
Cleaning the pipes.
Shout at your shoes.
Blow chunks.
Liquid burp.
Pray to the porcelain god.
Toss your cookies.
Sneeze cheese.
Lose your lunch.
Jazz up the carpet.
Eating backwards.
Shoot the cat.
Sing lunch.
Feed the fish.
Paint the back seat.
Goulash gush.
Call the whales.
Chow shower.
Bring it up for a vote.
The Call of the Walrus.
The liquid scream.
Jettisoning the chunky cargo.
Salad shooter.

Gut soup.
Yodeling groceries.
Heave up Jonah.
Whistle beef.
Call to the seals.
Speaking Dutch.
Review the menu.
Turn on the tap.
Throwing it into reverse.
Round trip meal ticket.
Spraying a jet.
Spray puree.
3-D burp.
Launching lunch.
Drive the bus.
Leggo my eggo.
Look for aardvarks.
Lose your load.
Toss the slack-macs.
Make a map.
Mouth crying.
Park the tiger.
Sing a rainbow.

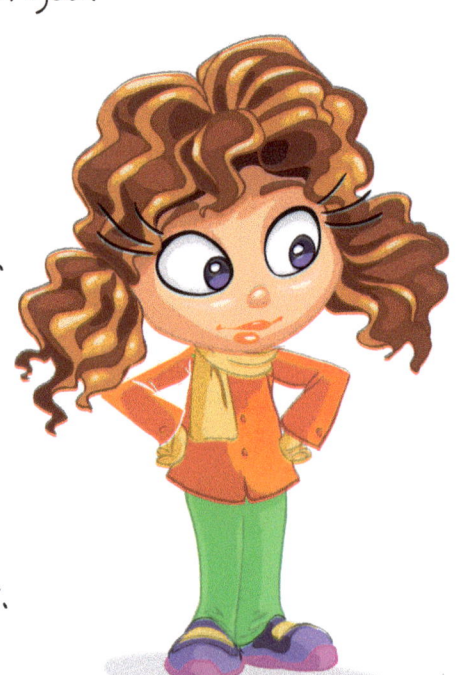

Spray the weeds.
Reverse peristalsis.
Doing the Hoakey Croaky.
Downloading dinner.
Arguing with the worms.
Esophogeal eruption.
Going for the second chew.
Fertilize the bushes.
Five finger spray.
Flash the hash.
Gastro geyser.
The big spit.
Oral diarrhea.
Hug the throne.
Paint the walls.
Honk smurfs.
Psychedelic yawn.
Sell the Buick.
Laugh at the ground.
Call for Huey.
Go the nostril sauce.
Call dinosaurs.
Acid chowder.
Rainbow kiss.
Bark at the ants.

Ride the regurgitron.
Rocket launching.
Spiff your biscuits.
Blow foam.
Drive a truck.
Playing the whale.
Liquidate your assets.
Big vom dot com.
Air one's paunch.
To cast up one's accounts.
Facial diarrhea.
Soul coughing.
Curl and hurl.
Out of stomach experience.
Quake one's gizzard.
Snot the hot dog.
Making your big toes go flat.
Spitting the furry lifesaver.
Smucking your yuck.
Growling splash monkey.
Blow grits.

5 POINTS FOR EVERY EXPRESSION YOU'VE HEARD.
100 POINTS WHEN YOU USE ONE IN A CONVERSATION.

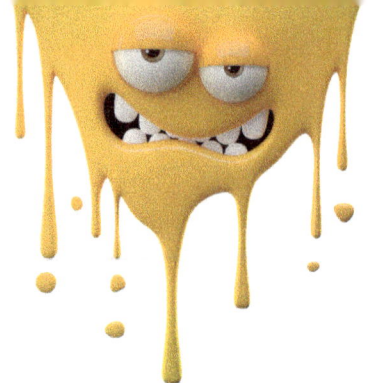

WHAT'S YOUR SCORE?

Page 2 First Burp	10 points (automatic)
Page 3 Mom's Memory	_____ points
Page 4 Burping Along	5 points (automatic)
Page 5 Quiet or Audible?	_____ points
Page 6 Burp Relief	_____ points
Page 7 Carbonated Burps	_____ points
Page 8 Animals and Parents	_____ points
Page 9 Ice Cream or Salad	_____ points
Page 10 Historical Burping	_____ points

Burping Subtotal _____

Page 13 Best Friend Belch	_____ points
Page 14 Girl Belch	_____ points
Page 15 Mom Belch	_____ points
Page 16 Class & Teacher Belches	_____ points
Page 17 Mouth Farts	_____ points

Belching Subtotal _____

Page 26 Funny Barfing?	_____ points
Page 27 Motion Sickness	_____ points
Page 29 Lovesick	_____ points
Page 32 Contagious Barfing	_____ points
Page 33 Snarfing	_____ points
Page 34 Not Barfing	_____ points
Page 35 Glossary	_____ points
Page 36 Old Words	_____ points
Page 37 Versatile words	_____ points
Page 38 Yelling Barf Sounds	_____ points
Page 39 Singing Barf Names	_____ points
Page 41 Barf Expressions	_____ points

Barfing Subtotal _____

Total Points _____

1-100 Angel – 101-999 Almost Normal – 1000+ Possible Psychopath

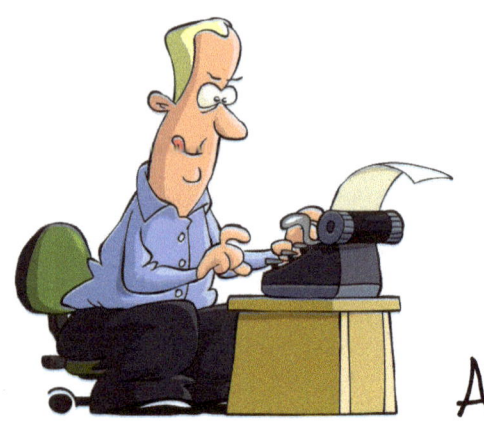

ABOUT THE AUTHOR

As an avowed burper, belcher, and sometime barfer, Jimmy Huston has studied these three subjects extensively and is considered an expert on two of the three. As a recovering screenwriter, however, he is not qualified to give advice on medical issues and certainly not on any matters of etiquette whatsoever.

Always well-behaved and above reproach, Mr. Huston totally disassociates himself from this book altogether. Unfortunately, he has written some other books, but they're no better and young readers should be discouraged from even opening them. (If you've already bought this book, he thanks you. If you haven't, do not read that last part yet.)

He grew up in Athens, Georgia, but now is allowed to live in Woodland Hills, California, with his future ex-wife and his dog. That's really all you need to know.

www.byjimmyhuston.com

Reviews are usually appreciated.

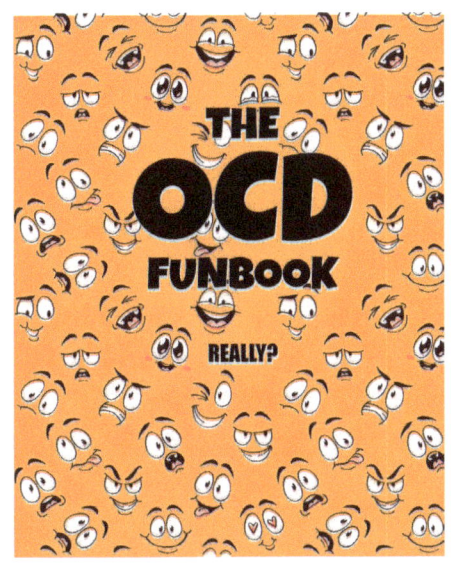
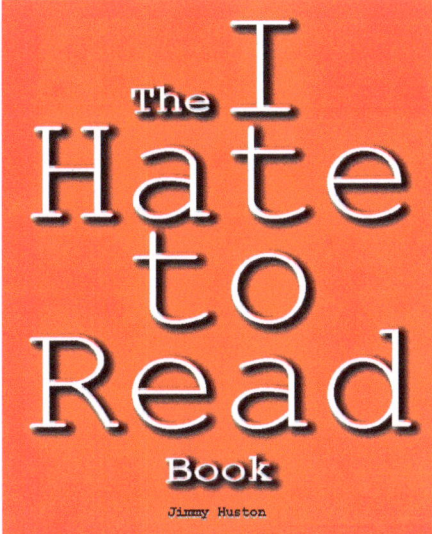
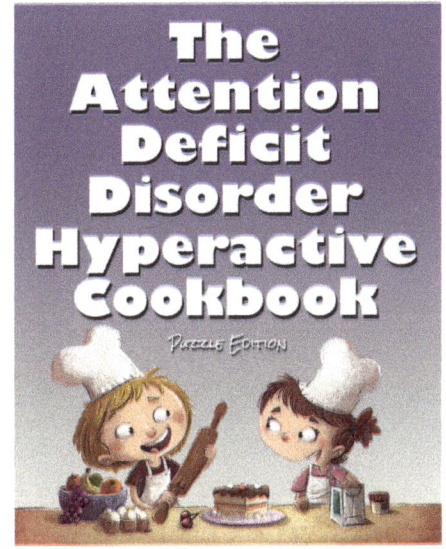

Other Books by Jimmy Huston

www.cosworthpublishing.com

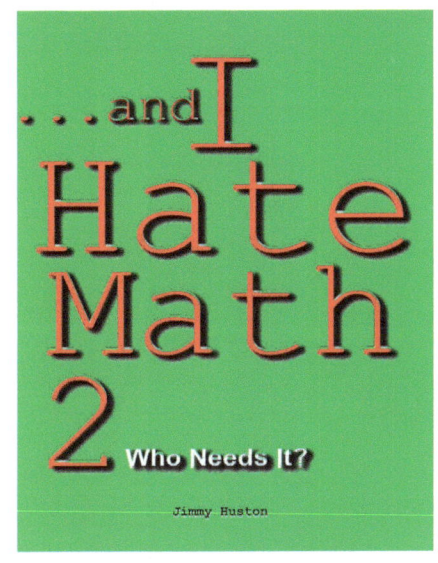
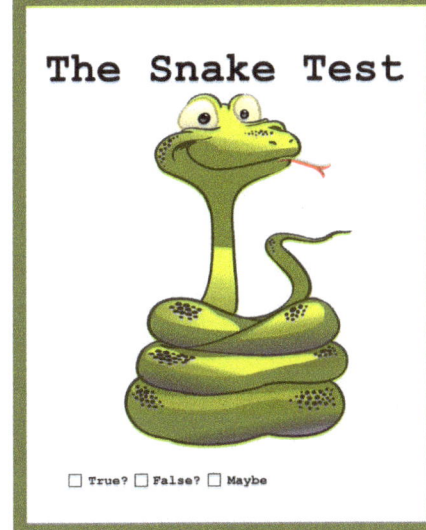
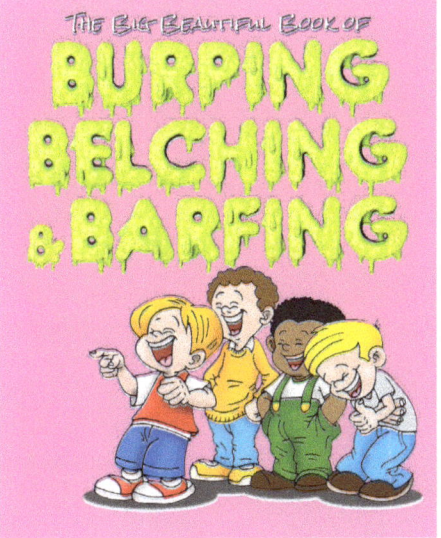
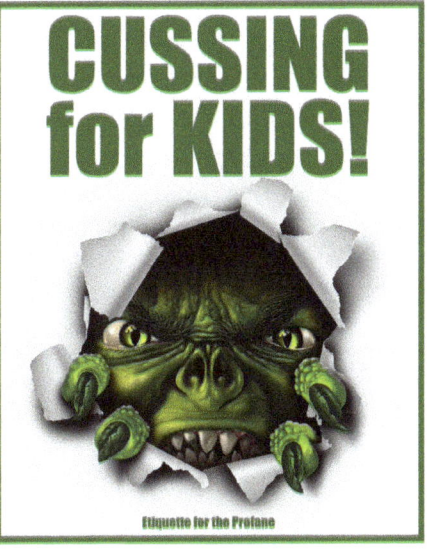

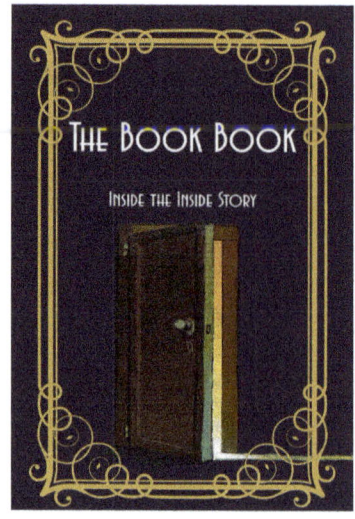
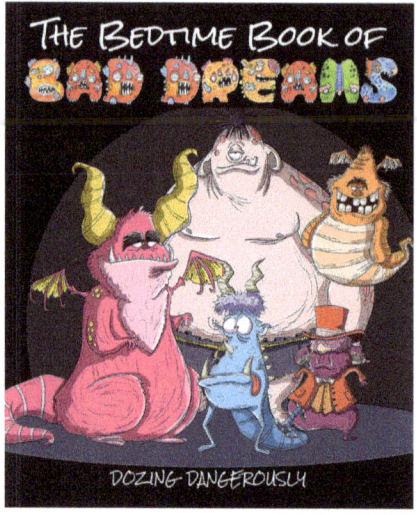
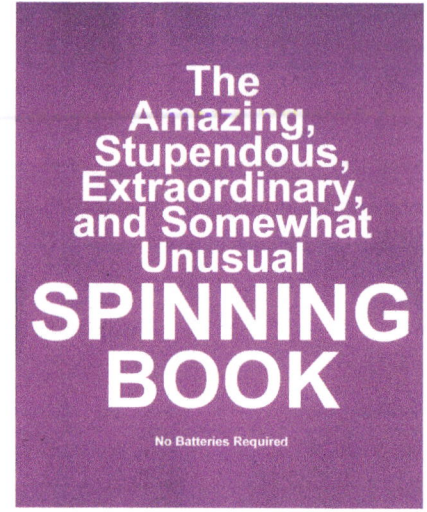
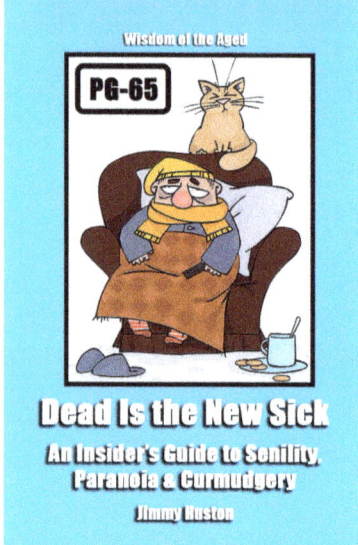

More Books from Jimmy Huston

www.cosworthpublishing.com

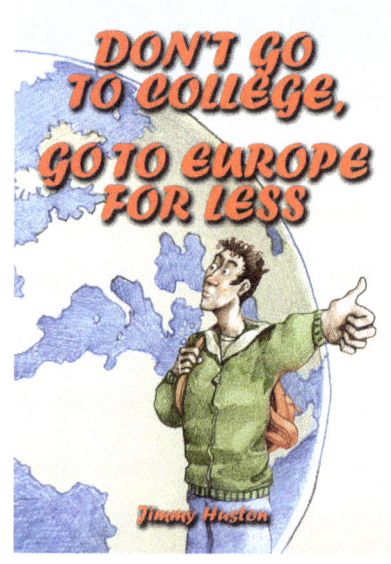
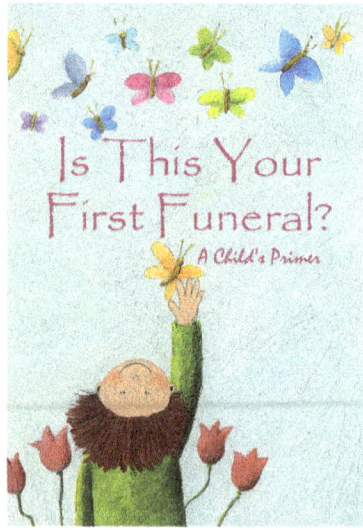
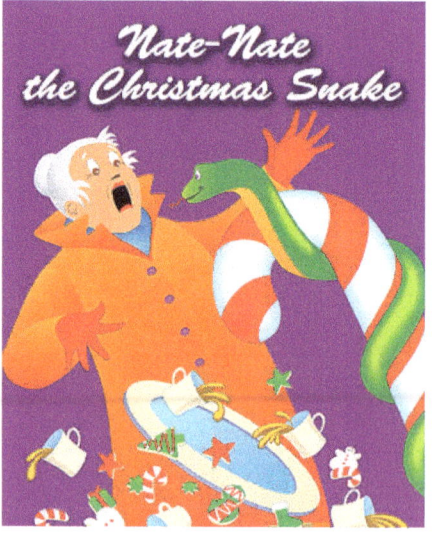
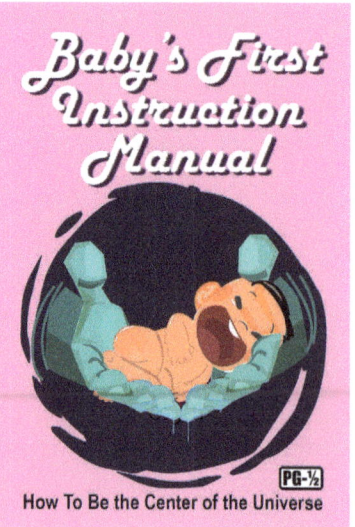

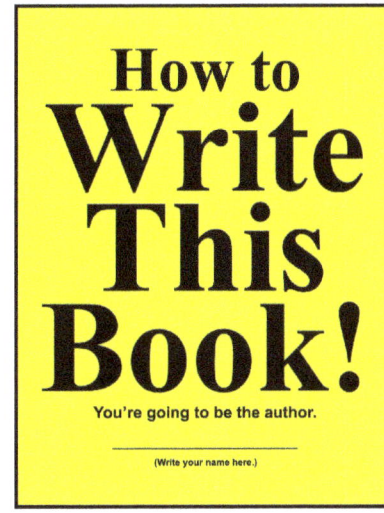
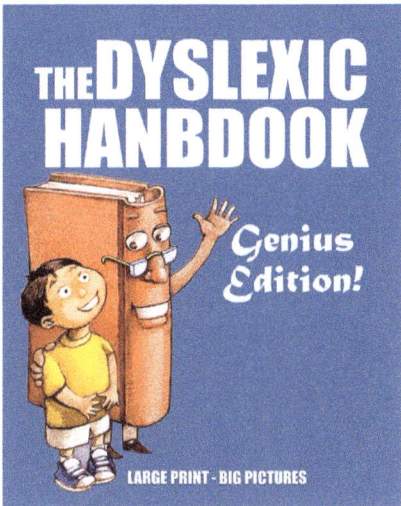
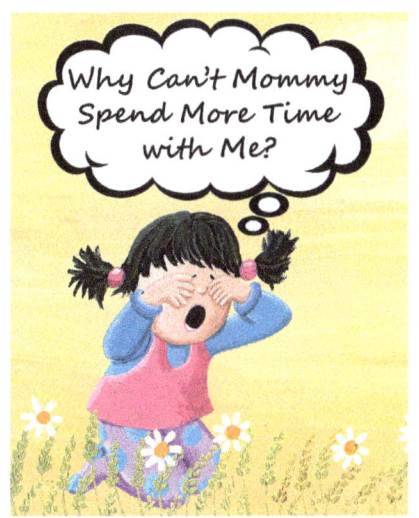
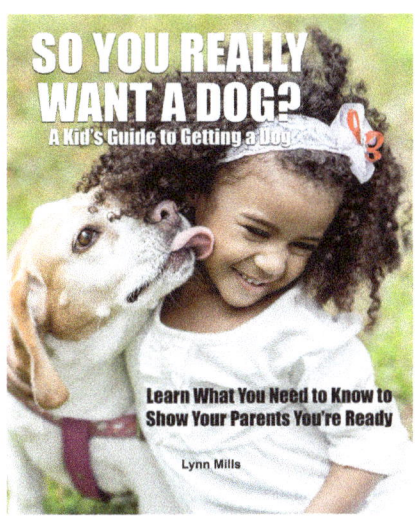

More Books from Cosworth Publishing
www.cosworthpublishing.com

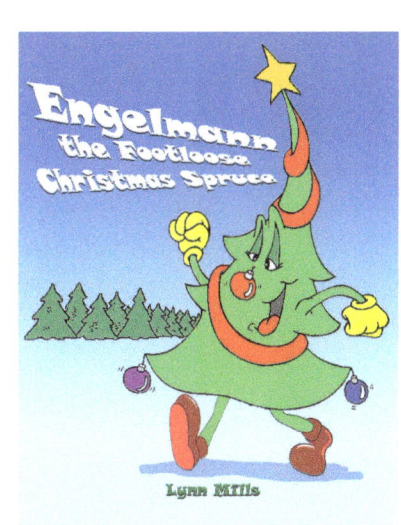
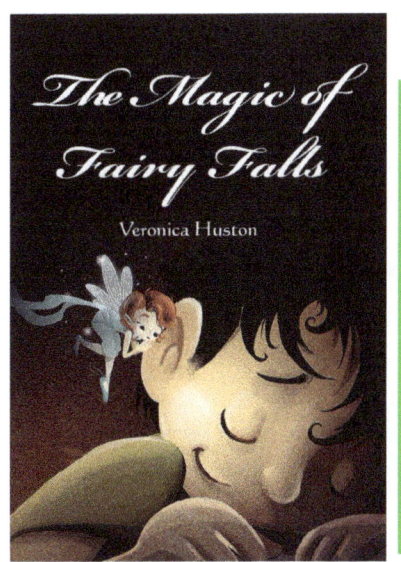
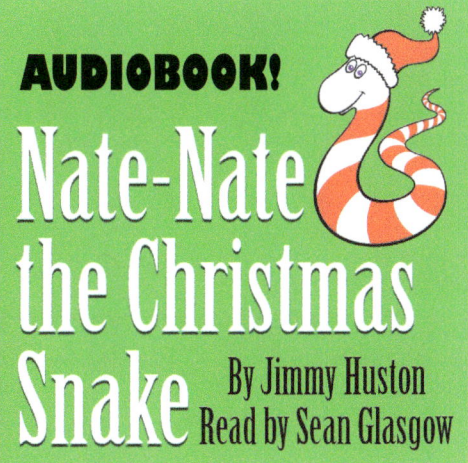
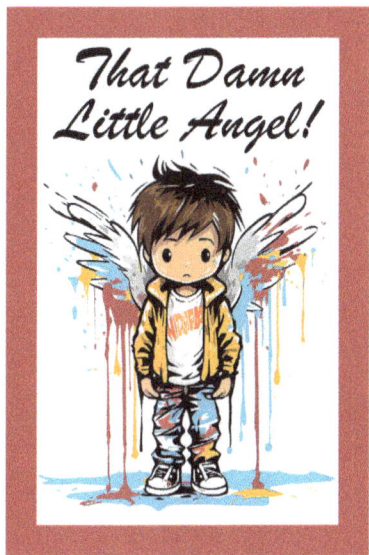

Books for Grownups from Cosworth Publishing
www.cosworthpublishing.com

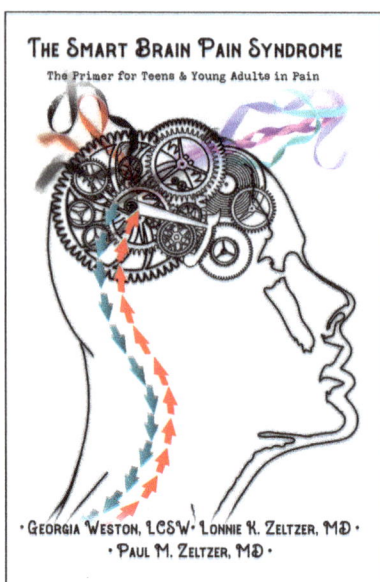

A groundbreaking new book. Three experts explain chronic pain to teens and parents, including using creative outlets to displace the pain.

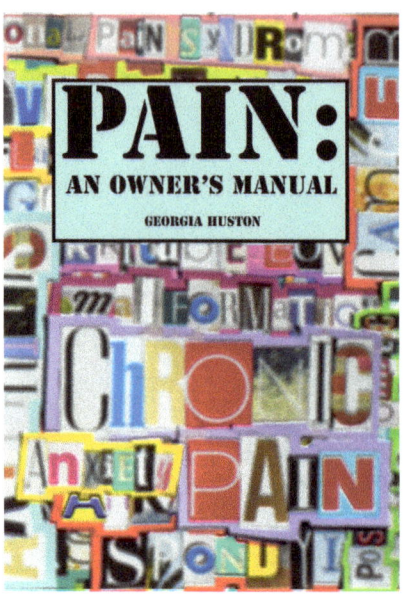

A young pain victim's inspirational and informative conversations with a variety of pain sufferers and specialists. Doctors should read this at their own risk.

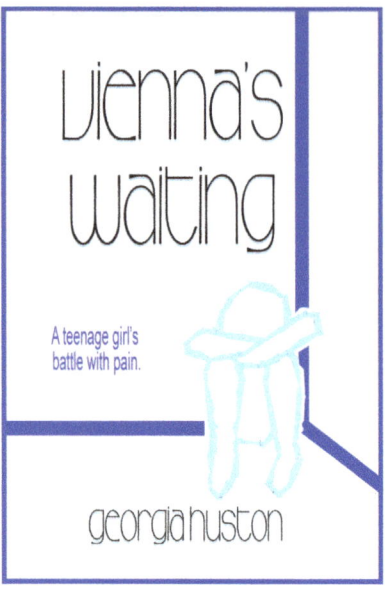

At 14, Georgia developed mysterious chronic pain. This book chronicles that dark time and follows her inspirational journey back to health and happiness.

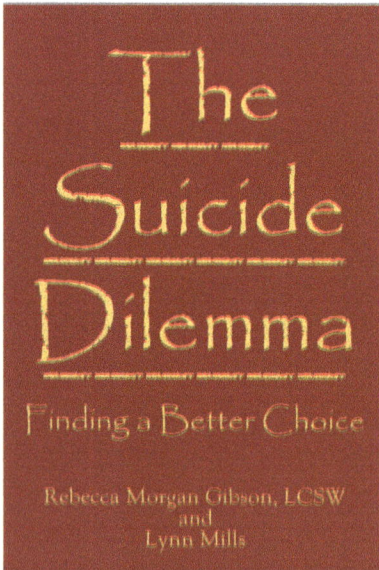

A practical guide for the person who is confronted by the possible suicide of a friend or family member.

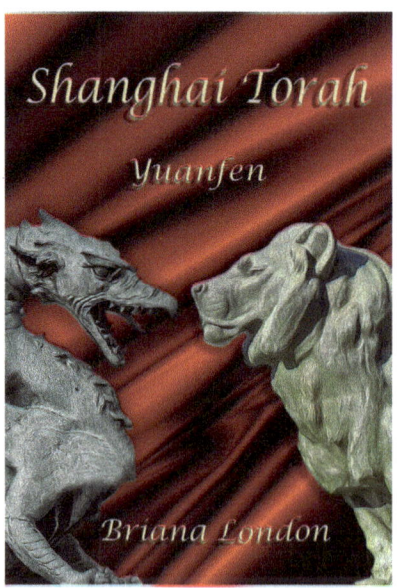

A young Jewish scribe flees WWII Europe with his in-progress Torah, escaping into China under Japanese occupation.

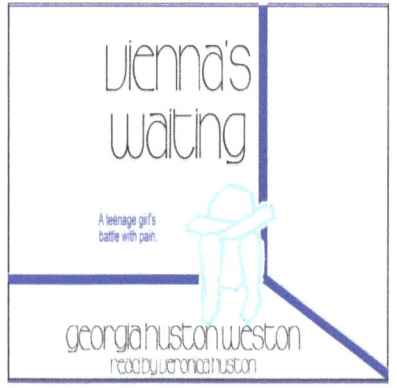

AUDIOBOOK

A powerful reading of Georgia's harrowing experiences as a young teen suffering chronic pain. Hearing it all out loud brings new power and meaning to this true-life story.

Thanks for buying, borrowing, or swiping this wonderful book.

At Cosworth Publishing we truly appreciate that, and in return, we'd like to offer you one of our E-books absolutely free—and worth every penny.

Just let us know that you want it, and we'll make sure that you get it. Let us know which book you read so we don't send you the same one.

Send an email to *office@cosworthpublishing.com*.

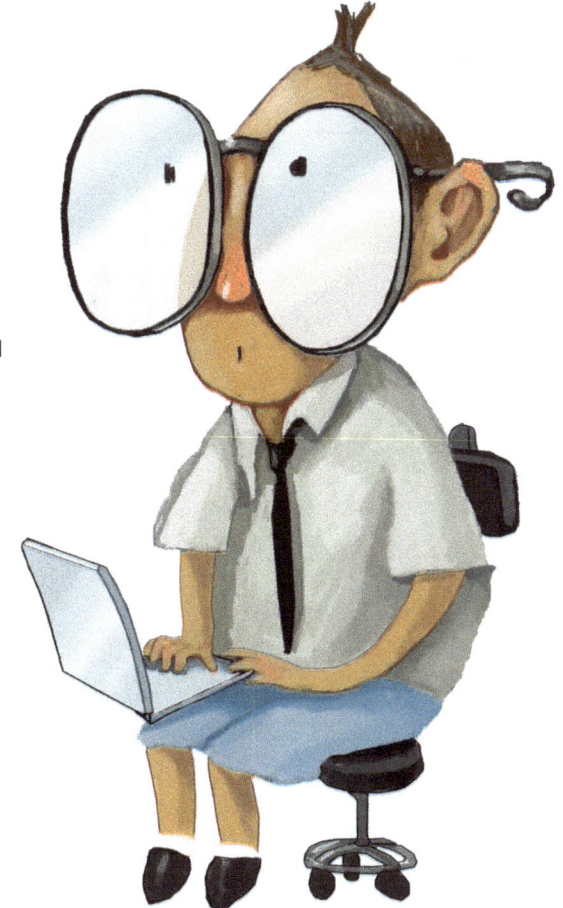

Then, from time to time, we will let you know via email when we have a new book that you might be interested in.

We won't do that very often because we're basically pretty lazy, and we don't produce very many new books.

Reviews are greatly appreciated.

www.ingramcontent.com/pod-product-compliance
Lightning Source LLC
Chambersburg PA
CBHW061114070526
44583CB00027B/3288